This book is dedicated to the 5.5 million women who read SELF magazine each month. Your quest to be your best keeps us striving to make SELF its very best.

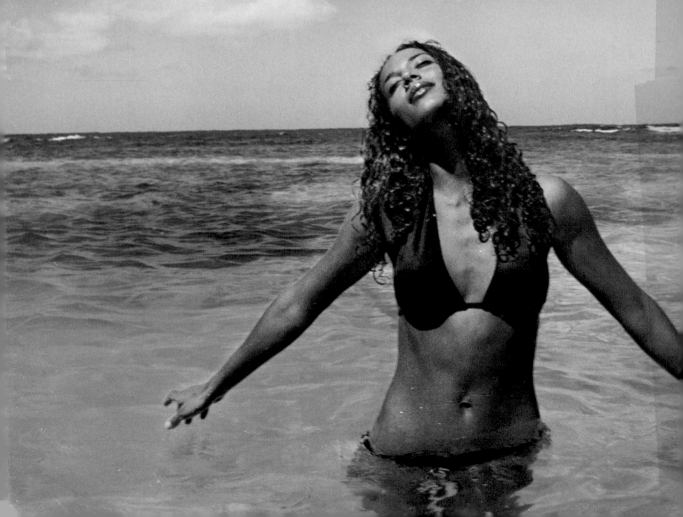

contents...

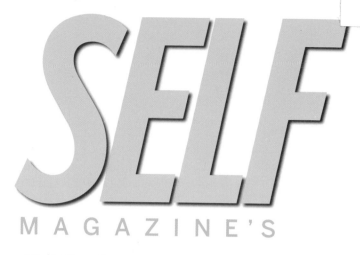

SELF
MAGAZINE'S
15 MINUTES TO YOUR BEST SELF

Quick fixes for a healthier, happier life

By Lucy S. Danziger and the editors of SELF

GOTHAM BOOKS

GOTHAM BOOKS

Published by Penguin Group (USA) Inc.
375 Hudson Street, New York, New York 10014, U.S.A.
Penguin Group (Canada), 90 Eglinton Avenue East, Suite 700, Toronto,
Ontario M4P 2Y3, Canada (a division of Pearson Penguin Canada Inc.);
Penguin Books Ltd, 80 Strand, London WC2R 0RL, England; Penguin Ireland,
25 St Stephen's Green, Dublin 2, Ireland (a division of Penguin Books Ltd);
Penguin Group (Australia), 250 Camberwell Road, Camberwell, Victoria 3124,
Australia (a division of Pearson Australia Group Pty Ltd); Penguin Books
India Pvt Ltd, 11 Community Centre, Panchsheel Park, New Delhi – 110 017,
India; Penguin Group (NZ), 67 Apollo Drive, Rosedale, North Shore 0632,
Auckland, New Zealand (a division of Pearson New Zealand Ltd);
Penguin Books (South Africa) (Pty) Ltd, 24 Sturdee Avenue, Rosebank,
Johannesburg 2196, South Africa

Penguin Books Ltd, Registered Offices:
80 Strand, London WC2R 0RL, England

Published by Gotham Books, a member of Penguin Group (USA) Inc.

First printing, January 2008
10 9 8 7 6 5 4 3 2 1

ISBN 978-1-592-40323-3

Printed in the United States of America

Designed by SELF Magazine

While the author has made every effort to provide accurate telephone
numbers and Internet addresses at the time of publication, neither
the publisher nor the author assumes any responsibility for errors or for
changes that occur after publication. Further, the publisher does not
have any control over and does not assume any responsibility for author
or third-party websites or their content.

Publisher's note: Neither the publisher nor the author is engaged in
rendering professional advice or services to the individual reader. The ideas,
procedures and suggestions contained in this book are not intended
as a substitute for consulting with your physician. All matters regarding
your health require medical supervision. Neither the author nor the
publisher shall be liable or responsible for any loss, injury or damage
allegedly arising from any information or suggestion in this book.

In my perfect world, I would exercise for an hour every day, and I'd have the body to show for it. I'd take my lunch hour—the full 60 minutes—outside, and after eating, I'd meditate or read a chapter of the latest best seller with the sun on my face. (I'd be wearing sunscreen with SPF 30, of course.) At 5 P.M. sharp, I'd make a clean break from the office, leaving my paperwork behind me. I'd ride my bike home to my well-behaved children, who would have already completed their homework. My husband would have the table set and a glass of wine poured for us.

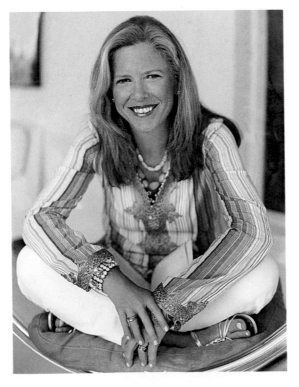

And I'd prepare a home-cooked meal. Or, better yet, he'd prepare it. Then, after dinner, we'd all play board games and laugh. My husband and I would put the kids to bed, have amazing sex and then fall asleep for a full eight hours on 800-thread-count sheets. We'd dream blissful dreams and awake full of energy and ideas.

Ah, to live a healthy, happy, well-balanced life. If only it were that easy.

Here's how my day usually unfolds: I wake up intending to jog a few miles, but if there's an early meeting, I skip the run. I down a cup of coffee, hustle the kids off to school—Where's the knapsack? Where's the field trip note?—and race into the office. Meetings, phone calls, more meetings. Oops, 3 P.M. and I missed lunch. Grab a salad at my desk. More meetings, then tear out of the door in time to oversee homework. Get home. Eat a few bites of the kids' leftovers. Help them finish their homework and get to sleep. Catch up on work by reading in bed, eyelids fluttering. Shut off the light and hope to get six hours of zzz's.

If being healthy and fit were an all-or-nothing proposition, most women I know, myself included, would be a lost cause. We haven't stopped caring about our well-being, certainly—we all want to be healthier, happier, fitter, prettier, better organized, more stylish and less stressed. We simply don't have time.

Women today are striving to stay one step ahead of the clock. But in trying to do it all, we often feel we don't do any of it well. There's no time to cook a healthy meal. No time to exercise, to get a checkup, to de-stress. According to a SELF survey of more than 2,000 women, 25 percent are too busy to take a single day off from work.

These sacrifices have put us on the fast track to health-and-happiness deprivation. Well, I say, Enough is enough. Let's put our own well-being atop our to do list. Even if it's only for 15 minutes a day. We all have 15 minutes, I feel certain. That's the time it takes to boil water and cook a pot of pasta, or take a shower and dry your hair.

Five years ago in SELF, we introduced a time-optimizing solution to our readers in a regular column called 15 Minutes to Your Best Self. It's a guide to the fastest, easiest ways to stay happy and healthy. Demand for more time-sensitive solutions grew so rapidly that we expanded 15 Minutes from a single page to three. I think the column is so popular because SELF solves our readers' time problems in a simple, fun, no-stress way. (Who has the time to devote an entire day, hour or life to being one's best? But 15 minutes? Who has time *not* to?)

As a magazine editor, I consider it a blessing when my staff and I hit upon a topic so useful that the hunger to read about it seems insatiable. To date, we've run dozens of 15 Minutes columns. But at the rate we're going, I will be 106 years old by the time we reveal all our great ideas. Why wait? That's why the talented group of writers, editors, researchers, photographers and design whizzes who put their all into SELF every month devoted themselves to bringing you a book packed with more of the surprising, smart, practical advice the magazine is famous for. If you can spend small pockets of time taking steps toward being your best self, the benefits will accumulate and your body, your mood and your life will change for the better. Try some of the 573 tips in this book, beginning today. The reward? A life that is brighter, healthier and more hopeful—all in 15 minutes a day.

LUCY S. DANZIGER, EDITOR-IN-CHIEF, *SELF*

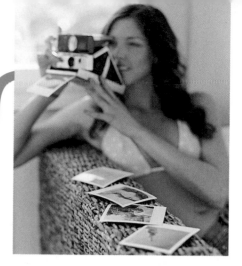

HOW TO USE THIS BOOK

On any given day, there are hundreds of ways you can improve your life in 15 minutes or less. But don't think of this book as a giant to do list. Rather, it's your tool kit for a better life. Open it when you feel like it. Put it away when you don't. If you're looking for help in a particular area of your life, dive into a specific chapter and work your way through it at your own pace. Dog-ear pages. Stick Post-its on your favorite tips. It's your book. It's your life. You have all the power to make it great!

YOUR PLEDGE FOR SUCCESS

Sign this contract as a reminder to take time out for yourself:
On _____, I decided that I would take at least a few minutes for myself every day. I pledge to stick with it because...
● If I don't make myself a top priority, no one else will.
● I feel happier when I am taking better care of myself.
● I believe that progress trumps perfection, and I know even baby steps can produce big results.

Signature

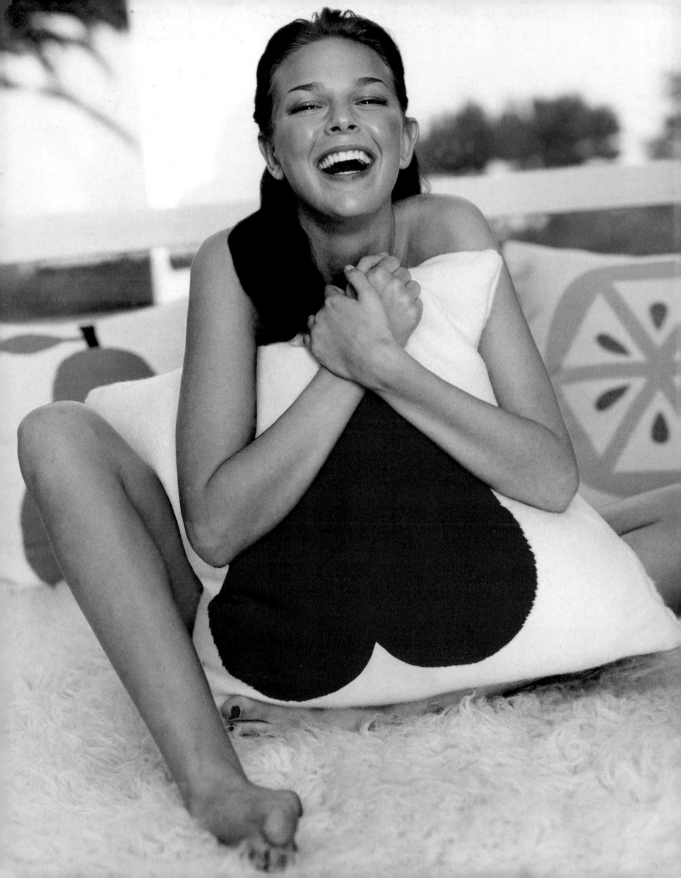

health improvers

Just think: In a matter of minutes and with minimal effort, you can significantly reduce your risk for heart disease, cancer, depression, Alzheimer's disease, infection and more. Simply turn the page to find a wealth of doable tricks and tips that can strengthen your health and lengthen your life. You get only one body, so why not show it some love? Taking care of yourself is easier than you ever thought possible.

The only 10 things you need to know to live a long, healthy and vibrant life

There are already so many ways to protect and heal our body, yet every day scientists seem to find even more stay-well strategies. Empowering? Yep! Overwhelming? Absolutely. Well, relax. Here, we cover the issues, weigh the medical research and simplify the essentials for you. The result is the mini insurance plan below.

1 Research your family history

Curiosity *can* save the cat: Knowing the specifics of your relatives' conditions will help you develop prevention strategies and reduce your risk for problems, including cancer, heart disease and depression. The info can also allow your M.D. to pinpoint the cause of certain symptoms. When you first approach your relatives for information, don't open with a personal question. Instead ask about the family in general and allow your relative to share her own history naturally, experts at the Mayo Clinic in Rochester, Minnesota, suggest.

2 Catch your zzz's

Too little pillow time is probably one of the greatest threats to your health, significantly raising your risk for heart disease, depression and weight gain. Some doctors say insufficient rest could be as devastating as poor nutrition or lack of exercise, says James B. Maas, Ph.D., professor of psychology at Cornell University in Ithaca, New York. "Your body uses sleep to restore itself, both physically and mentally," he says. While you're snoozing, it's hard at work repairing cell and tissue damage. So make like a log for seven to nine hours nightly. Easier said than done? Find a sleep specialist near you at SleepCenters.org.

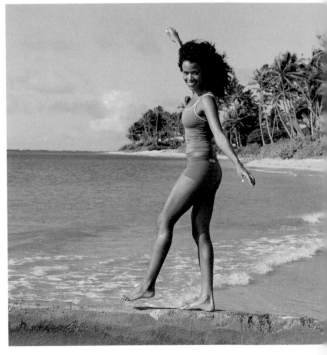

3 Bite right

Not only will making nutritious choices help you maintain a healthy weight, but by limiting your consumption of trans and saturated fats to 20 grams total per day (with as few trans fats as possible), you'll keep your body's level of inflammatory proteins low, which in turn maintains clear arteries. The flavonoids and antioxidants in fruit and veggies and the omega-3 fatty acids in fish and nuts can decrease DNA damage—which helps lower overall cancer risk.

4 Nix the butts

You know this, but we'll say it again: Smoking seriously raises your risk for heart disease and a range of cancers, including lung cancer, which kills more women every year than breast, ovarian and uterine cancers combined. Even if you're "only" a social smoker, it's still important to ask your doctor about a cessation aid such as nicotine-replacement therapy. Women appear to have greater success using two quit methods at once, so also check out the American Lung Association's Freedom From Smoking program at FFSOnline.org. And stay away from secondhand smoke; it's dangerous to everyone, regardless of who's puffing.

5 Soothe stress

When you're chronically frazzled, your brain increases production of stress hormones, which can damage cells over time. Stress might also contribute to high blood pressure, which nicks the arterial lining. Your body then repairs those nicks with cholesterol, and the buildup can contribute to heart attack and stroke. Your best bet? Create a stress-management strategy you can stick to: Pick a tension tamer such as yoga, or a social outlet that you enjoy, such as a cooking class, and blow off steam at least once a week. Also, have your blood pressure checked annually. If your systolic blood pressure (top number) is 120 or higher, step up the exercise. Cutting salt intake to less than 2,400 milligrams a day may also bring down that number.

6 Wear sunscreen

All sun exposure damages skin, and as little as 15 unprotected minutes each day could contribute to skin cancer (not to mention wrinkles). That's serious stuff. One in five Americans will get skin cancer, including melanoma, which accounts for the majority of skin cancer deaths. The rate of skin cancer has nearly tripled in women younger than 40 in the past 30 years. Slather on sunscreen every day, and use moisturizer and makeup with SPF.

7 Move it

Working out can help you stay at a healthy weight, which is crucial given that packing on excess pounds can increase blood pressure and cholesterol, and may lead to sleep deprivation, stress and depression, as well. Even if you're not overweight,

exercise (of the heart-pounding, heavy-breathing variety) has been shown to significantly lower the risk for heart disease, diabetes, Alzheimer's and cancer. Doing cardio or lifting weights for even half an hour a day is all it takes to reap big benefits, and any activity is better than none. Go to Self.com to try one of our simple fitness plans tailored to your body, your interests and your goals. You'll be amazed at how good you can look and feel.

8 Have safe sex

Unprotected sex can lead to HIV, human papillomavirus (HPV), hepatitis B and C, gonorrhea, syphilis, chlamydia and cervical cancer. Many of these diseases can impair fertility in addition to harming your general health. But don't be scared celibate. Always use a condom if you're unsure about your partner's status. The good news: Done the safe way, once-a-week nooky can improve immunity, and orgasms may even relieve migraines and menstrual symptoms. Feeling crampy? It's time to put on that Barry White album!

9 Take care of your pair

For women with no family history of breast cancer, the average lifetime odds of getting the disease are 1 in 13. Have your breasts examined by your doctor annually, and give yourself a once-over every month or so (see page 18 for instructions).

10 Buckle up!

Crashes are the leading cause of accidental death and injury for women ages 25 to 34 and the third overall killer (after cancer and heart disease) for those 35 to 44. Happily, seat belts save more lives than any other car-safety feature. So make a pledge: No matter where you sit or how short the trip, strap in every time.

◔ GOT 10 MINUTES? Figure out how healthy you are

Your answers to these questions will give you an objective view of your health and pinpoint a handful of minor changes that can have major health benefits.

1 How familiar are you with the medical history of your closest relatives?

- I know the medical histories of my parents and grandparents. +2
- I know the medical histories of my parents. +1
- I don't have a clue. 0

WHY WE ASK Although the history of your immediate family is most relevant to your health, knowing the specifics of your extended clan's health conditions can help you understand and even reduce your risk for problems, including breast cancer, heart disease and depression. The info can also allow your doctor to pinpoint the cause of symptoms more quickly. Keeping track is easy: Use My Family Portrait, a free tool available at www.hhs.gov/familyhistory. Taking control now means your family's health past doesn't have to be your future.

Your score _____

2 How regular are your periods (when you're not using hormonal contraception)?

- I have between 9 and 12 periods per year. +1
- I have about six per year. 0
- I have five or fewer per year. −1

WHY WE ASK "The menstrual cycle offers a window into a woman's health, including the status of bone health, cardiovascular health and ovarian health," says Paula J. Adams Hillard, M.D., professor of obstetrics, gynecology and pediatrics at the University of Cincinnati College of Medicine. Subtle changes can signal problems, and lack of a period is almost always a sign that something is out of balance. If you have very painful periods, prolonged heavy bleeding or few or no periods at all, talk to your doctor about what's going on.

Your score _____

3 When was your most recent Pap smear?

- Within the past two years +2
- Three or four years ago +1
- Five or more years ago −1

WHY WE ASK The Pap test is one of the best ways to prevent cervical cancer; it can detect up to 80 percent of abnormalities that lead to cancer, most of which can be treated quickly and easily. If you're 30 or older and have had three normal Paps in a row and no history of abnormal results, your gyno may allow you to have future screens every two to three years, as recommended by the American College of Obstetricians and Gynecologists in Washington, D.C. You don't get a pass on the pelvics, though—you should still have that physical exam annually to check for problems.

Your score _____

4 How often do you go to the dentist?

- At least every six months for cleanings +2
- Whenever I have a problem +1
- Almost never −1

WHY WE ASK If you make time for a cleaning and checkup regularly, you'll likely have fewer dental problems down the road, which can keep your body in better shape. To wit: Pregnant women who have gum disease may be seven times as likely to experience preterm labor. If you've fallen off the flossing wagon (or were never on), start small: Aim to do it every other day. Eventually, the habit will start to stick.

Your score _____

5 When was the last time you had your blood pressure and cholesterol checked?

- Within the past two years +2
- Several years ago +1
- I can't remember. −1

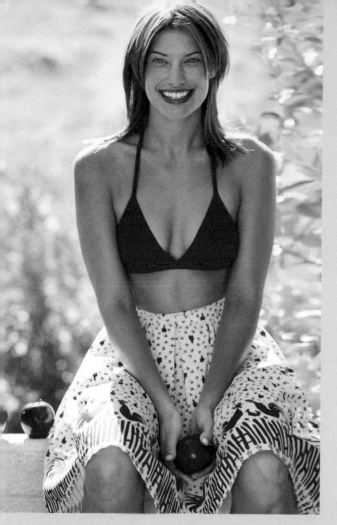

WHY WE ASK "Exercise not only improves the strength and function of your heart, circulatory system, muscles and bones, but it also helps you cope with stress and have a higher quality of life," says Cedric Bryant, Ph.D., chief science officer for the American Council on Exercise in San Diego. The best fitness programs combine cardio and strength training (e.g., running and lifting weights). If you need extra motivation, get step-by-step advice from Self.com.

Your score _____

7 What is your body-mass index? (If you don't know your BMI, see page 254 to calculate it.)

- Between 18.5 and 24.9 (normal) +2
- Between 25 and 29.9 (overweight) −1
- Below 18.5 (underweight) −2
- Thirty or higher (obese) −3

WHY WE ASK Your BMI can reveal important clues about your current and future health. For instance, being only 10 to 15 pounds overweight can raise your risk for diabetes, and losing that amount can bring your BMI back down. Research shows that people who have excess weight at middle age die earlier on average, often from heart disease, diabetes or cancer. Check with your doctor to make sure there aren't any medical causes behind your weight issue. If you need help getting in a healthy range, a registered dietitian can develop a meal plan. Find one at EatRight.org.

Your score _____

8 When was your last tetanus shot?

- Within the past 10 years +2
- When I was a child +1
- I've never had one, or I don't remember. 0

WHY WE ASK The Centers for Disease Control and Prevention in Atlanta recommends that all adults get the new Tdap vaccine, which protects against tetanus, diphtheria and whooping cough, if it has been more than 10 years since your last tetanus shots or if you often have close contact with infants. For more information on immunizations, visit CDC.gov.

Your score _____

WHY WE ASK Staying on top of your screenings can help you and your doctor monitor your risk for heart disease and determine whether you should be tested for diabetes. Get your blood pressure checked a minimum of once every two years and your cholesterol every five, assuming both are in the healthy range (below 120/80 for blood pressure and less than 200 milligrams per deciliter for total cholesterol). If your numbers are high, you can often lower them by improving your diet, exercising more or losing a few pounds.

Your score _____

6 How much sweat-inducing physical activity do you do each week?

- Thirty to 60 minutes most days +2
- Thirty minutes a few times per week +1
- Very little, if any −1

9 Which best describes your sexual practices?

- I'm in a long-term, mutually monogamous sexual relationship. +2
- I'm not committed to one person, but I always use condoms when I have intercourse. +1
- I'm not committed to one person, and I do not use condoms consistently. −5

WHY WE ASK Condoms are your best shot at protecting against HIV and a host of other sexually transmitted diseases, including chlamydia, gonorrhea and human papillomavirus (HPV), which each carry their own set of risks: infertility, ectopic pregnancy, cancer—the list goes on. That's why it's crucial to stay on top of your STD-screening tests, including the HIV test, which is now recommended for all sexually active adults.

Your score _____

10 How do you most often cope with stress?

- I regularly carve out time to recharge. +2
- I vent about my crises to friends or family. +1
- I don't. I just feel overwhelmed. −1
- I rely on drinking too much, overeating or indulging in another unhealthy habit to relax. −2

WHY WE ASK Frequent headaches, muscle tension and abdominal distress are all signs that it's time to make relaxation a priority. Schedule a massage, go for a walk, meditate for 10 to 15 minutes—whatever works. And if you still find that you have trouble unwinding without relying on risky habits, consider seeing a therapist. You can find one at APAHelpCenter.org.

Your score _____

11 How much alcohol do you drink?

- I average one drink or fewer per day. +1
- I occasionally have four or more drinks per night. −1
- I have about two drinks daily. −1
- I average more than two drinks a day; sometimes, I forget what I drank and what I did afterward. −3

WHY WE ASK Experts recommend that women have no more than an average of one drink a day and no more than three in a sitting. Exceed that and you're at increased risk for breast cancer, being in an accident (at home, outside or in a car), having unprotected sex or even being the victim of violence. If you tend to have a hard time applying the brakes in social situations, give yourself a drink limit (no more than two) before you head out for the night—and vow to stick to it.

Your score _____

12 Do you smoke?

- No, and I never have. +2
- I used to smoke, but I quit. +1
- I don't smoke, but I live with or work around smokers who puff near me. −3
- Yes, I light up regularly. −4

WHY WE ASK Simple: Smoking is the top preventable cause of heart disease, stroke and cancer. Which is why quitting is the very best thing you could ever do for your body. If you or a loved one need help kicking the habit, your doctor can help map out a quit plan, or you can visit QuitNet.com or BecomeAnEx.org.

Your score _____

13 Which of the following best describes your intake of calcium-rich foods such as lowfat dairy products or calcium-fortified OJ?

- I have three or more servings daily, or I take a calcium supplement [multivitamins don't count]. +2
- I have one or two servings per day. +1
- I have a few servings per week. −1
- I don't consume calcium-rich foods on a regular basis. −1

WHY WE ASK Women need 1,000 milligrams of calcium a day to protect against bone loss. All of the following contain between 300 and 350 mg of calcium: 1 cup nonfat or 1 percent milk; 1½ ounces reduced-fat cheddar, Jack or Swiss cheese; ¾ cup lowfat plain yogurt; 1 cup calcium-enriched OJ; 5 oz canned salmon with bones; and ¾ cup of certain calcium-enriched cereals, such as Total. Opting for a 500 mg supplement with vitamin D is a good way to fill any gaps.

Your score _____

14 How do you protect yourself from the sun?

- I slather on a moisturizer with an SPF of at least 15 every day and wear sunscreen when I'm outside. +2
- I don't wear block often, but I don't tan, either. 0
- I tan once or twice a year when I'm on vacation. –1
- I don't protect myself. I like to tan. –2

WHY WE ASK This simple step can slash your risk for skin cancer (the most common cancer in the United States), wrinkles and other signs of aging. Apply a healthy dose of sunscreen (a shot-glass full to cover your entire body) in the A.M., and if you're outside, reapply a minimum of every two hours. Choose products with at least an SPF of 30 that protects against both UVA and UVB rays. The ingredients to look for: titanium, zinc oxide, avoben-zone (also known as parsol 1789) and/or mexoryl. And to be safe, don't forget your hat.

Your score _____

15 How often do you use pain relievers?

- I take one once or twice a year. 0
- I use one occasionally. 0
- I pop a pain reliever most days. –1

WHY WE ASK Popping over-the-counter pain reliev-ers now and then is perfectly fine. But taking even the recommended dose of aspirin, acetaminophen or ibuprofen for too long may increase blood pressure, a study from the journal *Hypertension* finds. Compared with nonusers, women who took 500 mg or more of acetaminophen daily had twice the hypertension risk. Plus, other research has found that too much acet-aminophen may lead to liver damage, and overdoing it on aspirin and ibuprofen can contribute to ulcers.

Your score _____

YOUR TOTAL SCORE _____

How'd you do? Learn what your score means

20 AND HIGHER You're the picture of good health. Your only challenge is to keep up the great work. Stick to a regular exercise routine by treating yourself to a new pair of sneakers or some new tunes. Stay up-to-date on your checkups and immunizations with e-reminders at MyHealthTestReminder.com. And be sure to set aside at least 10 minutes a few times a day to decompress.

10 TO 19 You have some of the basics down, but other areas need your attention. Schedule a thorough checkup: If your ob/gyn is your primary doc, tell her that you're not seeing an internist so she knows to evaluate your health above the belt, too. Better yet, start seeing a primary care physician. Find out which diseases run in your family, then take steps to prevent them.

9 AND UNDER There is a lot of room for improvement. Set up a doctor visit pronto to catch up on screening tests, including those for HIV and other sexually transmitted diseases. Whether you need to slim down, shape up or quit smoking, set your sights on making

one good-for-you change in the coming weeks: Cut back on sugary snacks or take the stairs, say. Once you achieve that goal, tackle another. Every step counts if you're overweight; losing only 5 to 7 percent of your total weight can cut your risk for diabetes by 58 per-cent. Whatever your goal, you can do it!

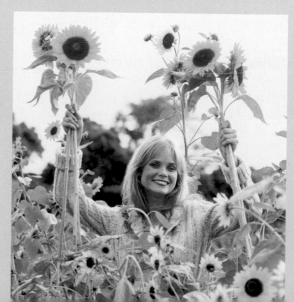

🕐 GOT 1 MINUTE?

Put your pillow to work Sleeping like a log may be easier than you think.

SIDE SLEEPERS Slip a pillow between bent knees to avoid back and hip pain.

BACK SNOOZERS Tuck a pillow under your knees or a rolled towel under the small of your back (or both) to gently relieve pressure on the spine.

HEADACHE SUFFERERS Consider the Chillow ($40; Soothsoft.com). Changes in pillow temperature may worsen pain. When filled with water, this foamlike pad stays cool. (It's encased, so it doesn't feel wet.)

SNIFFLE-AND-SNEEZERS Try one of the Personal Expressions Memory Foam pillows ($25 to $50; Sleep Innovations.com). Its special fibers thwart dust mites, and it's treated to cut down mold and allergen buildup.

STOMACH DREAMERS Skip the pillow underneath your head (it can strain the neck); instead, slide one under your pelvis and lower abs to ease pressure on the back. Settle in for sweet dreams!

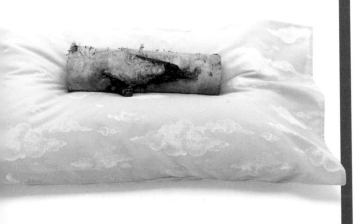

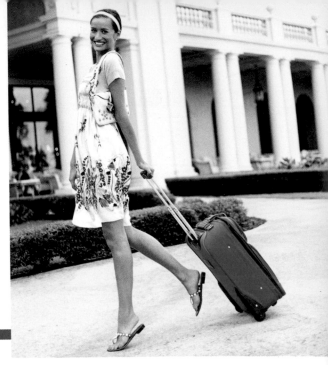

🕐 GOT 10 MINUTES?

Plan ahead to beat jet lag

HELP YOUR BODY get in sync with the local time, and nip jet lag in the bud, with these expert tips.

BEFORE YOU BOARD THE PLANE

Book an early flight. If you need to be in tip-top shape for a business meeting, bump up your arrival date. The extra time will give your body a chance to adjust.

Change your bedtime. Traveling east? Hit the sack one hour earlier starting a few days before departure. Going west? Stay up an hour for several nights in advance.

EN ROUTE

Sip smart. Drink plenty of water, and skip the in-flight cocktails. Lower levels of oxygen and increased cabin pressure cause you to feel the effects of alcohol more intensely, exacerbating the impact of changing time zones. Plus, who wants a hangover upon arrival?

AFTER YOU LAND

Stay awake. Keep yourself up until nighttime. A nap will only leave you awake when everyone else is asleep.

Slip on socks. At bedtime, warm feet will help your system slow down and ease you into slumberland.

Try melatonin. Popping a 3-milligram dose of melatonin about 30 minutes before bed can reestablish normal sleep patterns, says Candy Tsourounis, Pharm.D., associate professor of clinical pharmacy at the University of California at San Francisco. Warm milk also helps.

GOT 10 MINUTES?
Fend off insomnia

IF YOU WANT TO SLEEP but can't, or awaken hours too early, you may have insomnia. And because too few zzz's significantly raises your risk for heart disease, depression and weight gain, a healthy night's rest is crucial to your health. You can break the insomnia cycle for good with these surefire strategies.

Create a sanctuary. Draw the blinds, and turn on a fan or a CD of nature noises. Subtle, steady sound lulls you and blocks out distractions.

Leave the bedroom. If you find yourself tossing and turning, get up. Lying there stressing that you're awake will further rile your mind and body. Curl up with a boring book or do some relaxing but dull activity until you're drowsy, then head back to bed.

Set your alarm clock. Whatever time you finally close your eyes, get up at the same time every day (yes, even weekends). It may be painful at first, but the regularity will help your body relearn when it should be awake and when it should be asleep.

GOT 1 MINUTE?
Banish work from the bedroom

Associate your bed with sleep (and sex!), and you'll snooze more peacefully, according to the National Sleep Foundation in Washington, D.C. After all, who wants to sleep at the office?

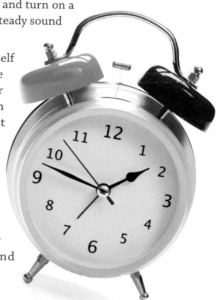

GOT 1 MINUTE?
Wake up refreshed

Throw a dark cloth over your alarm clock, if you have trouble drifting off. The glowing numbers can keep some people awake, the National Sleep Foundation notes.

GOT 5 MINUTES? Prepare for a sounder snooze

TAKE A LOAD OFF Calm an overly active mind by jotting down tomorrow's to do's before bed tonight.

SAY GOOD-NIGHT TO THE SCREEN The computer's light confuses your brain and makes it think it is daytime. Log off at least one hour before you hit the sack.

UNWIND WITH A PUZZLE Do Sudoku instead of sitting in bed with a scary novel. It's much easier to put down a game than to relinquish a gripping read.

🕐 GOT 4 MINUTES?
Do a breast check

PERFORM THESE STEPS with arms at your sides and again with each arm raised. You can explore your breasts either vertically from top to bottom or with small concentric circles from the nipple out—just choose a technique and stick with it. Do your checks every month or so; the goal is simply to know what's normal for you so you can spot something that is not.

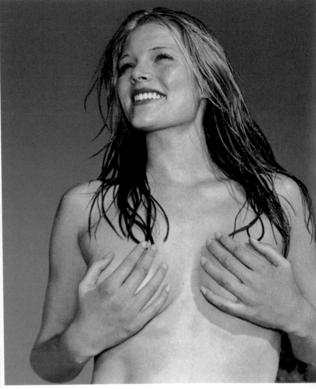

1 **Feel for lumps.** Imagine pressing on a bag of grapes: It may seem a bit lumpy in some areas (which is normal), but a small rock in the bag would stand out. Cancer rarely causes soreness, so pain in the absence of a lump is probably no cause for worry; but ask your doctor about anything that seems out of the norm.

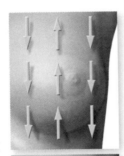

2 **Take a look.** Check for an inverted nipple, color changes, a rash or any discharge (particularly fluid that's brown, black or bloody). Any of these signs merits a call to a physician.

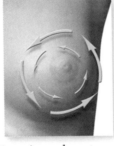

3 **Lie down.** With your breasts spread out, probe the region next to your armpit. If you feel lumpiness in one breast, check the other side. A bulge in the same location is probably nothing, but if it's new, contact your doctor.

4 **Scan your skin.** One kind of breast cancer that blocks lymphatic vessels can cause the skin to dimple so that it resembles an orange peel.

Extra credit After your doctor examines your breasts at your annual checkup, show her how you perform breast self-exams to make sure you're doing a thorough job. It's also a great opportunity to ask questions such as "So is this bump a normal lump?"

🕐 GOT 5 MINUTES?
Have some popcorn

Whole grains such as popcorn, rye and wheat are packed with fiber, which keeps you regular and may aid the body in eliminating excess estrogen that can stimulate the growth of breast cancer cells.

🕐 GOT 1 MINUTE?
Turn off *The Late Show*

Getting more shut-eye can protect your breasts. A study of 12,000 women in *Cancer Research* indicates that those who slept nine or more hours a night had a 72 percent lower risk of developing breast cancer compared with those who slept seven or eight hours. The more you snooze, the more melatonin you produce, which may help keep tumors from growing.

🕐 GOT 2 MINUTES? Let go of your fears

Discovering a lump in your breast can be terrifying. Before you panic, know that 80 percent end up being one of these benign conditions:

A CYST These fluid-filled masses are sometimes painful, but they rarely signal breast cancer and usually disappear on their own.

A FIBROCYSTIC CHANGE Monthly hormone fluctuation can trigger lots of mini-cysts and areas of thickened tissue throughout the breasts. An extra supportive bra can ease premenstrual soreness.

A FIBROADENOMA These solid lumps are especially common in young women. You can usually leave small ones alone, but you may want a large one removed so you won't worry every time you feel it.

🕐 GOT 5 MINUTES?
Schedule your screening

STARTING IN THEIR 20S, women should have their breasts examined during yearly checkups. The American Cancer Society in Atlanta recommends women 40 and older have annual mammograms. Women who have a mother or sister diagnosed with breast cancer before age 50 should have their first test at age 35 or 10 years before the age at which the relative was diagnosed, whichever comes first. And if you're at high risk (you have multiple relatives with the disease and/or have tested positive for one of the BRCA gene mutations), the ACS recommends an annual magnetic resonance imaging scan of the breasts, as well.

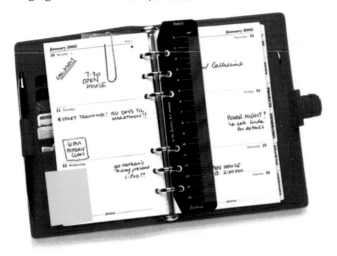

🕐 GOT 12 MINUTES?
Help find a cure

Want to give to a cause but not sure where to start? Find the worthiest breast cancer charities nationwide at CharityNavigator.org.

🕐 GOT 10 MINUTES?
Ask your dad an important question

For the fullest picture of your risk, look at your paternal family's health history, too. Consider aunts, uncles, cousins and grandparents as well as great aunts and uncles who had breast or ovarian cancer.

🕐 GOT 1 MINUTE?
Breathe clean air

Long-term, regular exposure to secondhand smoke may increase a nonsmoker's risk for breast cancer by as much as 27 percent, a review of 19 studies in the *International Journal of Cancer* notes. Plan your next girls night out at a cloud-free spot.

🕐 GOT 15 MINUTES?

Make a health date

These are the doctors you need to see and how often you should do so. Start scheduling now.

See your ob/gyn for

A Pap smear	**Every year until age 30** After 30 and three consecutive normal results, your doc may test you every two to three years.
A pelvic exam	**Annually** Your M.D. checks your vagina, uterus and ovaries. Ask about STD screening at this time.
A clinical breast exam	**Every year** Your ob/gyn should check your breasts at your annual pelvic-exam appointment.

See your dermatologist for

A clinical skin check	**Yearly** Your derm will scan for skin changes.

See your eye doctor for

An eye exam	**Every two years** Your doctor may suggest more frequent screening if you wear glasses or contacts.

See your primary care doctor for

A cholesterol test	**Every five years starting at 20** Get a breakdown of your HDL ("good"), LDL ("bad") and triglyceride levels.
A blood pressure test	**Your doctor may check at any visit.** Normal pressure is below 120/80.
A blood glucose screen	**Every three years starting at 45** If you are overweight or have a family history of diabetes, ask about starting screening sooner.

See your dentist for

An exam and cleaning	**Once or twice a year, depending on your doc** It's crucial to spot and treat gum disease as soon as possible; otherwise, it can increase your risk for heart disease.

🕐 GOT 1 MINUTE?

Don't wait for your doc

When you're making your appointments, ask for the first or last slot of the day. Patient traffic is usually lightest in the morning, and scheduling conflicts are often worked out by late afternoon.

🕐 GOT 2 MINUTES?

Know your medical rights

To get the treatment you deserve, exercise your right to...

● Have a copy of your medical records (so you can share with another physician or check for incorrect information).

● Request that a doctor rewrite a prescription if his handwriting isn't clear enough to read.

● Expect your physician to help you get a second opinion guilt-free, if you feel one is warranted.

● Refuse to be treated with products your doctor sells. Just because she profits from them doesn't mean you need them.

🕐 GOT 1 MINUTE?

Be prepared for emergencies

Make it easy for rescuers to reach your loved ones: Input your emergency contact info into your cell phone under the acronym ICE (in case of emergency). The paramedics will take it from there.

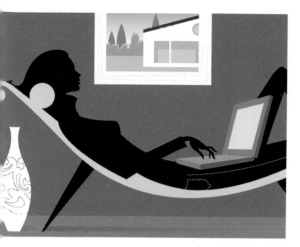

GOT 10 MINUTES?
Size up health info on the Web
Before you take online health advice, ask...

WHOSE SITE IS IT? Sites run by the government or a university are usually the most reliable. Check the editorial policy to be sure it has an advisory board made up of experts in the field.

WHOSE DATA IS IT? Medical statistics and facts should come from articles in established scientific journals; sources should be credited.

IS IT THE LATEST INFO? A site should indicate it has been updated recently. A lot of inactive links indicate that a site is not properly maintained and is likely out of date.

You can also make it easier on yourself by starting your search at a reliable comprehensive website. Four SELF magazine favorites:

- MedlinePlus.gov
- MayoClinic.com
- 4Woman.gov
- NIH.gov

GOT 5 MINUTES?
Avoid an M.D. mistake

STAYING INVOLVED in your care can prevent medical errors and improve outcomes. To be on top of things...

1 **Ask a friend to lend an ear.** Having a pal listen and take notes at an important appointment will help ensure you absorb all the information you hear.

2 **Arrive prepared.** Bring a written list of your questions, in order of priority. It will keep you from freezing up and forgetting your concerns.

3 **Keep 'em in the loop.** Be sure each of the doctors you see is aware of conditions being treated by other physicians, including what medication you're taking. Remember to share lab results, too.

4 **Be 100 percent honest.** Don't hold back on divulging not-so-healthy habits (smoking, drinking, unprotected sexual activity, drug use) or domestic violence. Your doc is there to help you, not judge you.

5 **Call for test results.** Lost lab reports are common. Don't assume your physician received yours.

6 **Trust your gut.** If you feel uncomfortable with a medical professional or your care for any reason, never hesitate to get a second opinion.

GOT 3 MINUTES?
Toss old drugs

Unlike over-the-counter medicines, prescriptions don't always list expiration dates. If a year has passed since an Rx was filled, it's time to throw it away; it may have lost some potency. Plus, you'll recoup shelf space.

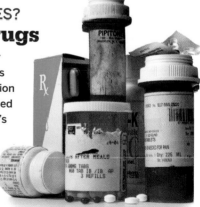

GOT 6 MINUTES? Copy your insurance card

Front and back. Stash the duplicates in your glove compartment and other purses so your information is handy in case you need it. Or commit your group number to memory so it's easier to look you up.

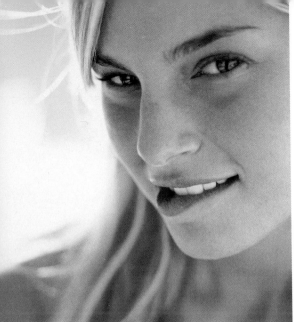

⏲ GOT 5 MINUTES?
Beat and treat colds and the flu

YOU CAN'T UNCATCH the viruses that cause cold and flu, but you can ease symptoms and maybe even knock a day or two off the course of your illness.

If you think you're coming down with a cold...

Try zinc lozenges. Research shows that zinc, particularly in lozenge form, can inhibit replication of the cold virus. Use it within 48 hours of symptom onset to shorten the duration or severity of your infection.

Turn down your air-conditioning. It dries the protective layer of mucus in your nose, which can prolong your suffering. If AC is a must, use an over-the-counter saline nasal spray to maintain moisture or sip chicken soup to hydrate and soothe throat inflammation.

HOW TO BEAT IT NEXT TIME Research shows that gargling with tepid tap water three times a day can wash away germs and reduce your chance of catching a cold by 36 percent. And wash your hands often, too.

If you think you're coming down with the flu...

Ask your doctor about antiviral medication. Prescription meds (specifically Tamiflu and Relenza) can slice a day off the length of your illness, as long as you take them within two days of your first symptoms. A day may not seem like much now, but when you're in the throes, any relief will be welcome.

HOW TO BEAT IT NEXT TIME Get a flu shot. You'll cut your chances of infection by 80 percent.

⏲ GOT 3 MINUTES?
Heal canker sores

Doctors don't know what brings on these mouth ouches, but they seem to form during times of fatigue and stress, when your immune system is run-down.

• To help soothe your inner cheeks and gums, mix 1 teaspoon each salt and baking soda in 1 cup water; swish four times a day.

• An over-the-counter treatment such as Kanka Mouth Pain Liquid can numb pain. In the meantime, go ahead and book that massage!

⏲ GOT 4 MINUTES? Get rid of a splinter

1 Gently wash the area around the splinter with soap and warm water, and swipe your tweezers with alcohol. Set them aside, and let them air-dry.

2 With clean, dry hands, sterilize a sewing needle by soaking it in alcohol a few seconds. Gently pierce the skin above the splinter, then use your tweezers to pull it free. (Don't dig around—if you can't easily extract it, leave it alone until you can see your doctor.)

3 After the splinter is out, apply a dab of antibiotic ointment and a bandage, and keep an eye open for signs of infection, such as redness, swelling or more pain.

🕐 GOT 1 MINUTE?
Protect your kisser

Up to 40 percent of us will get a cold sore, the American Academy of Dermatology in Schaumberg, Illinois, notes. These painful, contagious blisters are caused by the herpes virus (a different strain from the genital variety) and usually appear on the lips. Sun exposure can trigger an outbreak, so slather on a lip balm with an SPF of 15.

🕐 GOT 5 MINUTES?
Find relief from yeast

The signs of a yeast infection usually seem to be clear: a cottage cheese–like discharge and a serious urge to scratch. But before you self-treat with an OTC cure such as Monistat, see your doctor. Symptoms of vaginal infections can be similar, and it's critical to determine what you're dealing with because treatments often vary.

🕐 GOT 2 MINUTES?
Tackle tooth sensitivity

Overzealous brushing permanently weakens tooth enamel and separates gum tissue from the teeth, making nerves more susceptible to hot and cold. Use a loose, gentle grip; if you're still wincing through daily cleanings, consider switching to a sensitivity toothpaste such as Sensodyne.

🕐 GOT 2 MINUTES?
Conquer outdoor hazards Advice on handling three common alfresco pests

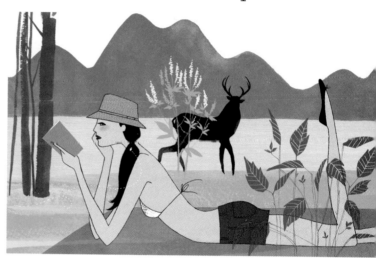

1 **SPOT POISON IVY** The plant abounds in gardens, so avoid anything that has leaves that grow in threes and turns red in the fall. If you do have a brush with the plant, "douse the area liberally with water, ideally within five minutes of being exposed," says Stephen Webster, M.D., a dermatologist in La Crosse, Wisconsin. Then wash your skin with laundry detergent for five minutes. Calamine lotion, antihistamines and oatmeal baths can ease the rash.

2 **SOOTHE BUG BITES** Don't scratch. Instead, apply an over-the-counter mentholated product such as Vicks VapoRub directly on the bite, says Neal Schultz, M.D., of Park Avenue Skin Care in New York City. "An itch is a low-grade form of pain," he says. "The brain can interpret only one sensation at a time, and cooling overrides itching."

3 **SCAN FOR TICKS** The ticks that cause Lyme disease, which initially triggers flulike symptoms (and sometimes a rash), are active in warm weather. After a day of summertime fun, do a full-body check. If you find one, use fine-tipped tweezers and grasp the tick as close to the skin as possible. Pull it straight out. Clean the area with soap and water. You may want to save the bug in a plastic bag so a lab, health department or even a vet can test it in case you develop any of the symptoms described above.

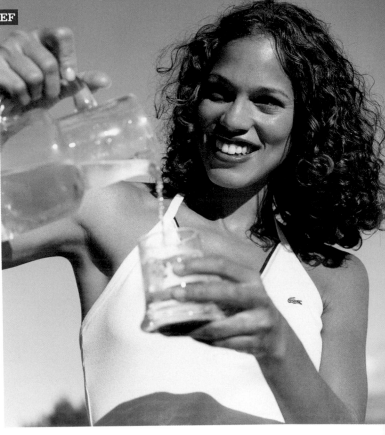

⏱ GOT 15 MINUTES?
Learn how to fight PMS

Keep a journal. The goal is to identify your personal pattern, so log your symptoms such as cramps, bloating, fatigue, headaches and the blues in a notebook. Mark when each occurs and rate its severity on a scale from 1 to 10. After two months, the pattern should be fairly obvious to you and your M.D. If your symptoms begin after you ovulate and end within a day or two of your period, PMS is likely to blame. If the same problems crop up all month long, your doctor can zero in on the right diagnosis.

Stock ibuprofen or naproxen. These over-the-counter pain relievers, known as nonsteroidal anti-inflammatory drugs (NSAIDs), can bring much-needed relief from cramps and even diarrhea.
- **For cramps** Pop naproxen starting the day before your period is due. It suppresses prostaglandins, the hormones that make your uterus painfully contract.
- **For diarrhea** Unfortunately, prostaglandins can have the same effect on your intestines as they do on your uterus. If you're prone, taking an NSAID before you typically get diarrhea can help keep you regular.

Lace up your sneakers. Working out can ease a whole range of PMS symptoms, including anxiety, mild depression, cramps, fatigue, bloating and irritability. In the short term, exercise kick-starts endorphin production, which can provide a temporary high. And over time, it helps normalize levels of the stress hormone cortisol, which has a lasting positive effect on mood. Try to break a sweat three times a week.

Eat almonds. If headaches crush you every month, consider increasing your intake of magnesium. Taking in 360 milligrams a day from foods such as almonds and pumpkin seeds can help ward them off.

Drink lots of water. It may seem counterintuitive, but the best way to deflate a bloated belly is to drink, drink, drink. Avoiding salty foods and getting at least 25 mg of fiber a day can help, too.

Plug in a heating pad. You can use an old-fashioned electric kind, but a self-heating adhesive patch can ease the ache for up to eight hours. A study in *Obstetrics & Gynecology* found that the pads can provide a level of relief similar to that of pain meds.

Consume calcium. Getting 1,200 mg of calcium a day, especially the week before your period, can improve mood. But for serious period-related depression, ask whether you're a candidate for an antidepressant. Certain ones can be highly effective when taken only during the second half of your cycle.

⏱ GOT 5 MINUTES?

Lift a low mood How to go from harried to happy

STRIKE A POSE Yoga is good medicine for your brain and your body. And cardio boosts the brain chemical serotonin, which helps you shake off life's stresses.

FLIP A SWITCH Some women are extremely sensitive to winter darkness. Counter the gloom by turning on a light box or going outside for 30 minutes each day.

JOIN A GROUP Research shows that social connections can help keep depression at bay. Becoming a member of an organization can help put problems in perspective.

EAT REGULARLY Having a little something to nosh on every three to four hours stabilizes hormone levels and your mood. Watch your alcohol and sugar intake, and make sure you have adequate amounts of protein and healthy fats in your diet.

⏱ GOT 2 MINUTES?

Mark your calendar

WE ALL FEEL down from time to time, but if your sadness persists for at least two weeks, it's a true disorder, says Eve Wood, M.D., clinical associate professor of medicine at the University of Arizona at Tucson. Talk to a therapist if your sadness is accompanied by these symptoms:

- Lack of motivation
- Appetite disturbance
- Concentration problems
- Unwarranted feelings of guilt
- Decreased sex drive

⏱ GOT 1 MINUTE?

Cheer for omega-3s

These unsaturated fatty acids target parts of the brain responsible for blue moods. Oily fish such as wild salmon and sardines are good dietary sources, but talk to your physician about taking a fish oil supplement.

⏱ GOT 10 MINUTES?

Shed the stigma

Dealing with depression is nothing to be ashamed about.
KNOW THAT YOU'RE NOT ALONE One in 10 people suffers from depression every year, and women are twice as likely as men to develop it. In fact, a woman is more likely to develop the condition than to be diagnosed with breast cancer.
SHARE YOUR SADNESS Confiding in someone about your sad spell beats bucking up alone. Let your family, friends or a therapist help you through your tough times and you will rebound much more quickly. And if you recently had a baby, reaching out for support is especially important. Pregnancy causes hormonal shifts that can leave new moms vulnerable. Talk with your doctor if you're feeling overwhelmed.

⏱ GOT 4 MINUTES?

Watch for relapse

Nearly half of patients with depression suffer only one episode. But if you're hit again, there's a 75 percent chance you will have a third. After that, the likelihood of recurrences goes up. If you've had three episodes, talk to your doctor about long-term antidepressant therapy.

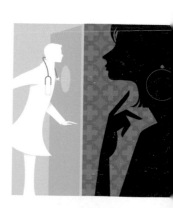

⏱ GOT 5 MINUTES? Pinpoint the source of your stomach woes

A sharp stabbing on the right, a dull ache lower down, general queasiness—there are as many types of tummy pain as there are causes. Find out what's ailing you.

IT'S PROBABLY	IF	WHAT TO DO
Acid reflux	• You have pain in your upper abdomen at least twice a week. • You also experience a burning sensation under your breastbone.	**If the pain strikes only once in a while,** try chewable antacids or OTC acid reducers such as Zantac. But when flare-ups occur more than twice a week, you're probably possessed by gastroesophageal reflux disease, which tends to be chronic. Call your M.D. for an exorcism (usually prescription-strength meds with a few lifestyle changes).
Constipation	• Your pain pops up after you eat. • You haven't had a bowel movement in a few days.	**To get things moving,** try a laxative or stool softener. To prevent future bottlenecks, drink plenty of water, maintain a steady exercise routine and gradually up your fiber intake to 25 grams of fiber a day with whole grains, beans, fruit and veggies or a fiber additive such as Citrucel.
Food poisoning	• Your discomfort develops within a few hours of eating. • You also experience diarrhea, nausea and/or vomiting.	**Just sit tight** and allow your body to rid itself of the toxins. Skip anti-diarrheal medicines so your body can expel what it needs to. If you can keep anything down, sip clear liquids, especially sports drinks, to prevent dehydration. If you're still throwing up or having diarrhea after a day or you develop a fever, call your doctor right away.
Irritable bowel syndrome	• You experience frequent pain in your lower abdomen. • You have a change in your bowel habits but no other symptoms.	**Keep track of your symptoms,** as well as what you ate and what was going on in your life to determine triggers. Then share your log with your physician, who can help you create a treatment plan that may include prescription medications, psychotherapy, hypnosis, antidepressants, diet changes and/or an exercise regimen.
Lactose intolerance	• You have pain in your lower abdomen at least once a week. • Your symptoms occur only with dairy.	**Try this home test.** Eat little or no dairy for two weeks; if the symptoms disappear, you're likely lactose-intolerant. Try eating small quantities of your favorite dairy foods with a lactase enzyme supplement. But to reach your 1,000 milligrams a day of calcium, you may need a supplement.
An ulcer	• You get a sharp pain in your upper abdomen at least once a week. • You start to feel better after eating.	**See your doctor to confirm.** These sores in the stomach lining are usually triggered by a bacterium that typically lies dormant for years. Your physician can detect it through a blood test. If the test is positive, you'll get a round of antibiotics and several months' worth of an acid-reducing medication such as Prilosec to help the ulcer heal.

GOT 15 MINUTES?

Exercise away stomach upset

Who knew? Moving the area where your legs and hips meet activates your intestines, easing constipation and gas. Good equipment bets: the StairMaster and elliptical trainer. Don't have time for the gym? Try a simple abdominal massage. Press three fingers near the right hip; slide them up toward ribs, then across and down.

GOT 30 SECONDS?

Cool heartburn

Chew fruit-flavored gum to produce acid-neutralizing saliva, says Stuart Spechler, M.D., of the University of Texas Southwestern Medical Center at Dallas.

GOT 1 MINUTE?

Defeat the bloat

A few extra crunches along with sitting up straight may be all you need to keep bloating in check. That is because women often feel inflated in the late afternoon, when abdominal muscles slacken, which allows food to expand into a greater space, explains Lawrence Brandt, M.D., chief of gastroenterology at Montefiore Medical Center in Bronx, New York.

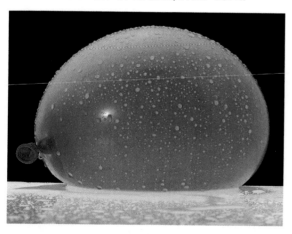

GOT 1 MINUTE?

Sip smartly to ease constipation

Chilled beverages tend to slow down digestion. To keep things moving along, have water or tea at room temperature.

GOT 10 MINUTES?

Take a belly breather

Stress and nervousness can cause diarrhea as easily as food can. A relaxing stroll can soothe your belly and mind.

🕐 GOT 15 MINUTES?
Buy a new vacuum

Regular cleaning is necessary to control nagging household allergens such as dust mites and pet dander, but your efforts can be detrimental if you use the wrong vacuum. Many vacuums are inefficient because they suck up the allergen and then spit it right back out into the air through the bag. Pet dander in particular is extremely small and can fit through the tiny holes in vacuum bags. Your best bet: Buy a vacuum with a HEPA (high-efficiency particulate air) filter, which can trap the particles inside.

🕐 GOT 1 MINUTE?
Learn if you have a cold or allergies

Wondering why you've been sneezing? Compare these lists.

YOU PROBABLY HAVE A COLD IF...
- You have a low-grade fever.
- You have thick, discolored mucus.
- You're unusually fatigued.
- Others around you are sick.
- Your symptoms develop within three days of being exposed.
- You feel better and more like yourself in five to seven days.

YOU LIKELY HAVE ALLERGIES IF...
- You don't have a temperature.
- The mucus you have is clear and runny.
- No one around you is sick.
- Symptoms develop after contact with an allergen or at the same time every year.
- Symptoms last as long as your exposure to the allergen.

🕐 GOT 8 MINUTES?
Kill mold fast

Mix 10 parts water and 1 part bleach in a spray bottle and mist the infested area. Leave for five minutes—any less and you may not kill the mold—then wipe clean with a disposable rag. Finally, vacuum the area, because when mold dies, it sheds a sneeze-prompting substance that can accumulate in house dust.

🕐 GOT 6 MINUTES?
Kick kitty dander

MOST ALLERGISTS AGREE that the best way to fight cat allergies is to get rid of the pet. If you can't bear to, limit her to certain areas of your home. Keep bedroom doors shut, and block out the main living area. Dander can stick around for up to a year after the animal is removed, so don't expect immediate results. For even more control, wipe down your cat with a wet cloth once a week to absorb dander. Better yet, have someone else rub down Fluffy for you so you're not exposed.

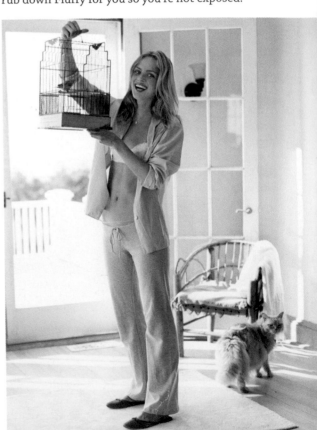

🕐 GOT 5 MINUTES?
Avoid allergy triggers Sniffle-inducing substances can lurk in some unusual places.

SUSPECT	WHAT HAPPENS	THE CURE
Fido	Pollen attached to your furry friend could send you sneezing.	Bathe him weekly, and on high-pollen days, wipe his coat with a wet cloth before allowing him to come indoors.
Your pillow	The filling may harbor up to 16 types of allergy-triggering fungi, research from the University of Manchester in England shows.	Wash synthetic pillows in hot water every three months and cover all your pillows with allergy-proof cases. (You can find them at most bedding stores.)
Your houseplants	Fuzzy growths or black stains on the leaves are an obvious sign of a dreaded allergy trigger: mold.	Wipe off spots, and keep plants near a window so they stay dry. Don't overwater. Toss the pot if you can't get rid of the mold.

🕐 GOT 10 MINUTES?
Zap a flare-up

Visit the drugstore for an over-the-counter med with loratadine—it will clear your allergies up without conking you out. Need something stronger? A prescription-strength antihistamine or a steroid nasal spray may be in order. Check in with your doctor.

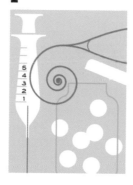

🕐 GOT 5 MINUTES?
Map out your personal prevention plan

STOP ALLERGIES before they start with this checklist:

- Note where you are when symptoms occur.
- Make an investment in allergen-blocking covers for your mattress, pillows and duvet.
- Shut your windows when pollen counts are high. Check the count at Pollen.com.
- Change the filter in your air conditioner and/or run an air purifier in your bedroom to help clear the air.
- Clean your home: Vacuum, disinfect the bathroom and wash your sheets once a week.

🕐 GOT 2 MINUTES?
Strip the bed

The bane of many an allergy sufferer's existence is the microscopic dust mite, which lives in carpets, pillows and bedding and is nearly impossible to eradicate completely. But washing your bedding in at least 140-degree water can kill the bugs, experts from Yonsei University in Seoul, South Korea, say.

🕐 GOT 6 MINUTES?
Wash your hair

Kick allergy triggers out of bed: Scrub your scalp before you hit the sack to get rid of the allergens that have latched on to your strands during the day.

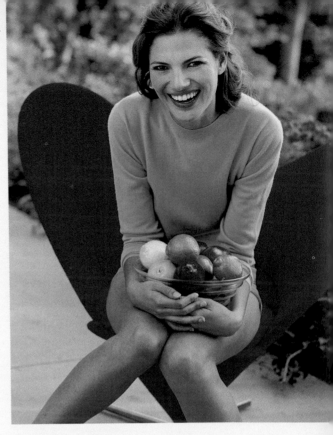

⏱ GOT 15 MINUTES?

Assess your heart health

Only one in four women can accurately predict her own heart disease risk, a SELF survey notes. Learn where you stand by answering the questions below.

1 How old are you?

Younger than 40   –5   Older than 55   +10
40 to 55 years old   +7

Your score _____

2 Is one or both of your parents African American?

Yes, and you're younger than 40   +2   No   0
Yes, and you're 40 or older   +1

Your score _____

3 Do you get at least 30 minutes of sweat-inducing, heart-pumping exercise six or seven days a week?

Yes   –1   No   +1

Your score _____

4 Where does most of the fat in your diet come from?

Primarily from foods such as olive oil, nuts, olives, avocados and soft trans fat–free margarine   –1
Mostly from foods such as meats, cheese, whole milk, margarine and ice cream   +1

Your score _____

5 Do you already have coronary heart (aka coronary artery) disease, blood vessel narrowing, diabetes or chronic kidney disease, or have you ever had a stroke?

Yes to any   +20   No   0

Your score _____

6 Do you smoke one or more cigarettes a day?

No (Jump to question 8)   0
Yes, and you're younger than 50   +9
Yes, and you're older than 50   +4

Your score _____

7 If you answered yes to question 6, do you also take oral contraceptives?

Yes, and you're younger than 35   +5   No   0
Yes, and you're 35 or older   +10

Your score _____

8 Do you have a borderline high blood glucose level, or have you had gestational diabetes?

Yes   +10   No   0

Your score _____

9 Has your father or a brother had a heart attack before age 55 and/or has your mother or sister had one before age 65?

Yes   +2   No   0

Your score _____

10 Do you tend to become overly stressed, fly off the handle when you're upset or allow negative feelings to smolder?

Yes +1   No −1

Your score _____

11 Have you ever had depression for longer than four years (treated or untreated)?

Yes +1   No 0

Your score _____

12 Were you overweight or physically inactive as a kid, or did you weigh less than five pounds at birth?

Yes to any +1   No 0

Your score _____

13 Do you eat at least nine servings (or 4½ cups) of colorful fruit and vegetables every day?

Yes −1   No 0

Your score _____

14 Do you floss your teeth daily?

Yes −1   No 0

Your score _____

15 Your waist is

35 inches or greater +2   Less than 35 inches 0

Your score _____

16 Your total cholesterol score is

Less than 200 milligrams per deciliter 0
Between 200 and 240 mg/dL and you're
    Younger than 50 +8   50 or older +4
Greater than 240 mg/dL and you're
    Younger than 50 +10   50 or older +7
You don't know your cholesterol and you're
    Younger than 50 +9   50 or older +5

Your score _____

17 Your HDL ("good") cholesterol is

Less than 50 mg/dL +2   Greater than 65 mg/dL −1
Don't know +2   50 to 64 mg/dL 0

Your score _____

18 Your triglycerides are

150 mg/dL or greater +1   Don't know +1
Less than 150 mg/dL 0

Your score _____

19 Your systolic blood pressure (the top number) is

You don't know +3   150 or greater +4
Between 130 and 149 +2   Between 120 and 129 0
Less than 119 −1
If you take blood pressure medication, add an extra +2

Your score _____

YOUR OVERALL SCORE _____

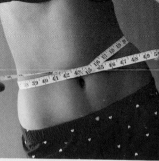

What your score means

LESS THAN 9 You're at very low risk and seem to be doing everything right. Keep up that healthy lifestyle!
FROM 9 TO 19 You're at low risk for heart disease. Review the quiz to ID potentially problematic behaviors, and turn the page for tips on staying in a healthy range.
FROM 20 TO 22 You're at moderate risk, so it's time to start making healthy changes in your life. The biggies: Exercise, eat a lowfat diet and seek help for depression, if you have it. Also, if you're a smoker, chuck your cigarettes once and for all. Finally, see your family doctor for a comprehensive checkup and custom plan.

GREATER THAN 22 You're at high risk. Schedule a complete exam with your doctor ASAP. The sooner you start making healthy lifestyle changes, the bigger the impact you're likely to have on your own heart health.

SELF thanks Debra R. Judelson, M.D., director of the Women's Heart Institute at the Cardiovascular Medical Group of Southern California in Beverly Hills, for developing this assessment, and Orli R. Etingin, M.D., director of the Iris Cantor Women's Health Center at New York Weill Cornell Medical Center in New York City, who helped with the editing and scoring. This quiz is based on the 10-year cardiovascular risk calculator, available at www.nhlbi.nih.gov/guidelines/cholesterol.

◔ GOT 10 MINUTES?

Reduce your cardiac risk Regular exercise and avoiding smoking are important. But so are these lesser-known strategies. Try one or more today!

Ban trans fats. If saturated fat is bad, then trans fat is downright ugly. This man-made substance (found in most anything fried, processed or commercially baked) increases the production of LDL ("bad") cholesterol in the liver, which over time starts to cling to artery walls, forming plaque. The more it builds up, the narrower your arteries become, which raises your risk for high blood pressure, stroke and heart attack. Ditch trans fats and instead load up on foods rich in omega-3 fatty acids, such as salmon, or a fiber-filled veggie stir fry, which help keep arteries clear so blood can zip along.

Take the blues seriously. If you're feeling depressed, your heart may be suffering. Studies suggest that higher amounts of stress hormones in depressed people raise blood pressure and increase inflammation. What's more, the lethargy that often accompanies the condition can keep a person from sticking with heart-helping habits. If you're suffering, ask your doctor for a referral to a therapist.

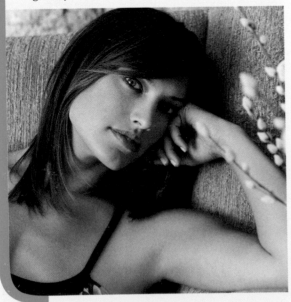

Request a blood sugar test. Diabetes is such a strong risk factor for heart disease that doctors treat their diabetic patients as if they already have cardiac trouble. One possible reason why: People with high blood sugar often have high levels of insulin, which can cause small arteries to become dysfunctional. Routine screening doesn't start until age 45, but you might need a blood test sooner if you meet any of the following criteria: You have high blood pressure; elevated total cholesterol or elevated LDL cholesterol; high triglycerides or a waist larger than 35 inches; you're overweight, have polycystic ovary syndrome or a history of gestational diabetes; or you're African American or Hispanic. The number-one way to cut your chances of developing diabetes in the first place? Drop some of the extra pounds (if you have them). Losing merely 5 percent of your body weight can make a significant difference in your overall risk.

Check your own pressure. Your doctor probably measures your blood pressure at every office visit, but you can do it yourself, too, at many pharmacies. Anything below 120/80 is considered healthy. The reason to watch it? The higher your pressure, the harder your heart has to work to pump blood throughout the body. If left untreated, it can lead to not only heart attack but also stroke, kidney problems and vision loss. The best ways to keep it low: Exercise, maintain a healthy weight, avoid cigarettes and watch your salt intake.

Assess your numbers. If you have no clue what your cholesterol levels are, it's time to schedule your test. The healthy limits: Your total cholesterol should be below 200 mg/dL. Your HDL ("good") cholesterol should be 50 mg/dL or higher. Your LDL ("bad") levels should be below 150 mg/dL; and your triglycerides, the most common fat in the body, should be below 150 mg/dL.

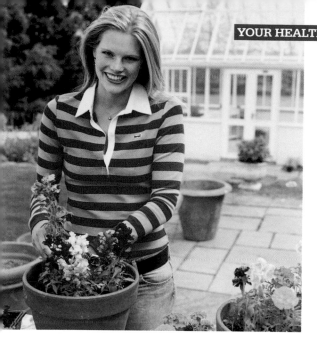

⏱ GOT 10 MINUTES?
Slow down

WOMEN WHO RACE through the day are twice as likely as their tortoiselike counterparts to develop high blood pressure, a study from Northwestern University in Chicago suggests. Use these two tricks to ease out of the fast lane:

SCHEDULE DOWNTIME Block out 10 minutes a couple of times each day to simply relax. Breathe deeply, do yoga, knit. Consider it a health investment, not wasted time.

CHECK YOUR SPEED When you catch yourself rushing through something, stop and ask yourself whether you truly need to be in such a hurry. To promote a more measured pace, stop, breathe deeply and count slowly to 10 when you're moving from one project to another.

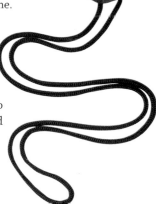

⏱ GOT 5 MINUTES?
Dig in for a happy heart

Here's a dirty little secret: Cultivating a garden is a proven stress reliever. Researchers at New York University in New York City found that people who spent time gardening in a greenhouse had significantly lower heart rates than those who didn't exercise their green thumb. Spend five minutes potting a plant, and you could benefit, too.

⏱ GOT 1 MINUTE? Learn how to spot a heart attack

You may think the signs of a heart attack would be obvious—crushing chest pain, trouble breathing—but they may be more subtle, especially in women, according to the American Heart Association in Dallas. If you or a loved one experience any one of the following, call for an ambulance immediately.

- Chest pressure. This sensation may feel like fullness or outright pain in the middle of the chest. It may be continuous, or it may come and go.
- Discomfort in the upper body. One or both arms may be affected as well as the back, neck, jaw or stomach.
- Shortness of breath. Patients may experience some trouble breathing; it may or may not be accompanied by chest pain.
- Nausea, feeling dizzy or breaking out in a cold sweat

⏱ GOT 10 MINUTES?

Build a sense-saving kit
Damage to your senses can happen right under your nose. In fact, it can start accumulating as early as your 20s. To help ensure that your senses continue to provide the info (and pleasure!) you deserve, pick up these sense-protecting essentials:

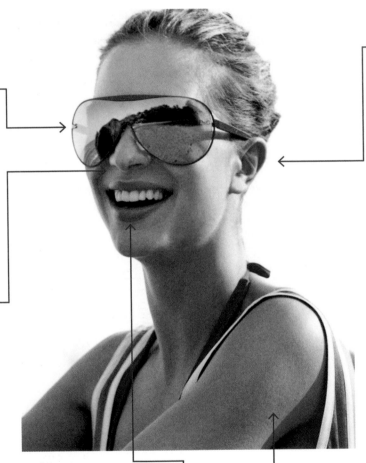

A pair of sunglasses to help you stay clear-eyed

Make sure they have at least 99 percent UV protection. Look for the American Optometric Association seal.

Saline spray to safeguard your nose

Cold and flu viruses can wipe out nasal nerve cells, eventually dulling your sense of smell. Keep your nose moist with a saline spray, especially in dry weather; it will discourage bacteria from taking hold.

Ear plugs to buffer your ears

Once the hair cells that detect sound waves are destroyed by loud noise, they're gone for good. (Used frequently, even a mower or a blender can cause hearing damage.) When it's noisy, use foam ear plugs, says Mary Florentine, Ph.D., Matthews Distinguished Professor at the Institute for Hearing, Speech and Language at Northeastern University in Boston. You'll enjoy sweet sounds for years to come.

A tongue scraper to boost flavor

Gently cleaning your tongue may help remove bacteria colonies as well as open up your taste buds. It may also help change the composition of saliva so that more food dissolves, intensifying flavor.

Moisturizer to power your touch

Dry skin can weaken and slow touch signals en route to your nerve endings. Moisturize, and don't overexfoliate; the irritation could dampen sensitivity more.

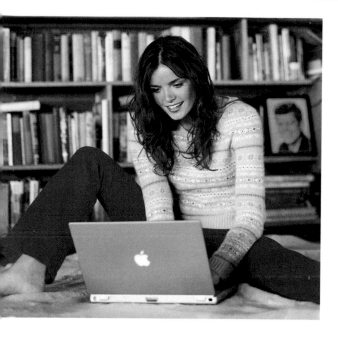

⊕ GOT 1 MINUTE?
Pamper your peepers

Spending hours on your computer can cause eyestrain, marked by burning, dryness or irritation. That's because blinking lubricates the eye, and you do it less while you're staring at the screen. Worse, if you squint while you surf, you'll blink even less. To help protect your eyes, simply blink more often and dim overhead lights to minimize any glare.

⊕ GOT 1 MINUTE?
Test your hearing

RUB YOUR THUMB and index finger together, an inch away from one ear, then the other. If the sound is much softer on one side, you may have an infection, a blockage or even early hearing loss. Consider getting a full evaluation, especially if hearing loss runs in your family. And keep the sound on your MP3 player and TV below a third of the maximum volume; if the guy next to you is grooving to your tunes, you've got it cranked up far too high.

⊕ GOT 1 MINUTE?
ID an infection

Lightly tap your cheeks, forehead and between your brows. If you feel pain and pressure, you could have a sinus infection. Call your doctor stat!

⊕ GOT 3 MINUTES?
Fix a feast for your eyes

Leafy green veggies are rich in the antioxidant lutein, which may reduce the risk for cataracts and age-related macular degeneration. Add spinach, kale or broccoli to your sandwiches, soups and salads for an eye-opening bite.

GOT 30 SECONDS?
Keep whites pearly
Attention, soda sippers: Down your drink with a straw angled toward the back of the mouth. This little move can help reduce your chance of tooth decay.

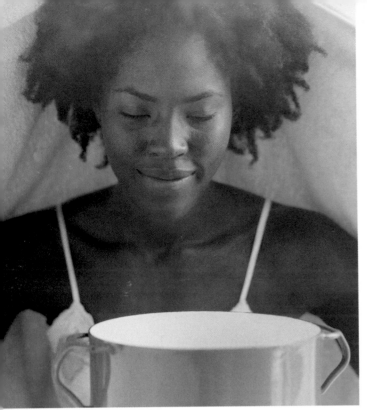

GOT 8 MINUTES?
Steam away sinus troubles

If you're congested, headachy or feel feverish, it might be the beginnings of a sinus infection. Boil a few white onions. Breathing in the stinky steam with your head under a towel for several minutes can help open stuffed-up nasal passages, plus onions have proven antiviral properties. (Add beef broth, and you're halfway to French onion soup!)

GOT 1 MINUTE?
Add spice to your morning

Sprinkle cinnamon on your oatmeal and latte. Research published in *Diabetes Care* found that consuming as little as ¼ teaspoon of the brown powder daily helped reduce blood sugar levels in people with type 2 diabetes. Cinnamon, which has insulin-enhancing compounds, also lowered triglyceride, LDL cholesterol and total cholesterol levels.

GOT 1 MINUTE?
Mend cuts with honey

Honey can disinfect wounds and help them heal faster. It contains an enzyme that produces hydrogen peroxide, which kills germs, and its antioxidants may also reduce inflammation. (Raw honey is most effective, but a dab from your bear will work.) Warm the sticky stuff in the microwave, apply a tablespoon to a gauze pad and secure with medical tape. Reapply daily.

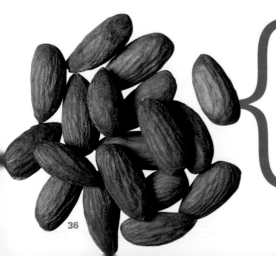

GOT 3 MINUTES?
Go nuts for heart health

GRAB A SMALL HANDFUL of nuts, especially walnuts or almonds, and crunch your way to lower cholesterol and blood pressure. Nuts are high in heart-healthy monounsaturated fat and omega-3 fatty acids, which help reduce LDL ("bad") cholesterol and keep the walls of the arteries healthy and elastic. Just be sure to stick to a small portion—1 ounce of nuts (about 23 almonds) contains between 160 and 200 calories.

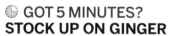

⏱ GOT 1 MINUTE?
NIP BAD BREATH IN THE BUD

The cinnamon-flavored chewing gum Wrigley's Big Red reduced bad-breath-inducing bacteria by more than 50 percent, according to researchers at the University of Illinois at Chicago.

⏱ GOT 5 MINUTES?
STOCK UP ON GINGER

You may reach for ginger ale to soothe tummy trouble, but you'll get more relief from the real deal. Opt for ginger tea, capsules or fresh ginger (in soup).

⏱ GOT 2 MINUTES?
SAVE YOUR STOMACH

Love sushi? Don't skip the wasabi. There's a reason your rolls come with this sinus-clearing green paste: Japanese horseradish has antibacterial properties that can help prevent food poisoning.

⏱ GOT 6 MINUTES?
HAVE A CUP OF TEA TO FEND OFF CANCER

Drinking at least two cups of green or black tea a day may cut your risk for ovarian cancer by nearly half. Both brews are rich in cancer-fighting antioxidants, which can help protect reproductive cells.

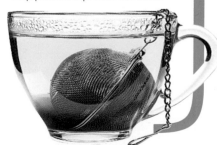

⏱ GOT 2 MINUTES?
Wake up when you're behind the wheel

Put a drop of peppermint essential oil on a tissue, and inhale the scent while you're stuck in traffic or on a long drive. Getting a whiff can help make you more alert and decrease frustration.

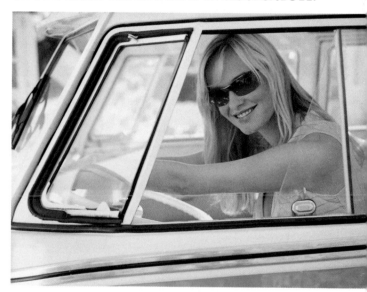

⏱ GOT 15 MINUTES?
Thwart a UTI

Susceptible to urinary tract infections? Drinking 16 ounces of cranberry juice a day can ward them off. The fruit keeps E. coli, the bacterium that causes most UTIs, from sticking to the wall of the bladder, making it harder for infection to take hold. Once you have a UTI, it's too late for cranberry juice—the red beverage can't kill the bacteria. Call your doctor and ask for a prescription for an antibiotic instead.

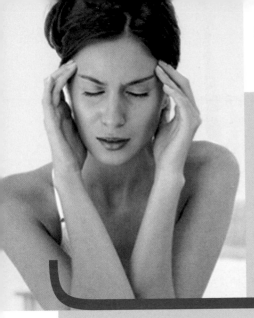

⏱ GOT 2 MINUTES?

Figure out if it's a tension headache or a migraine

Almost every woman is bound to get a headache this year. And though 75 percent of the pains are related to tension, nearly 20 million women suffer from migraines as well. Use these detection strategies to learn which one you're prone to and how to get relief.

It's probably tension if

You feel a dull, pressing pain on both sides of your head. Muscle tightness is the usual cause.

HEAD IT OFF
- **Take a computer break every 30 minutes,** says Allan Bernstein, M.D., chief of neurology at Kaiser Permanente in Santa Rosa, California.
- **Check your posture.** The main sensory nerve in your forehead is rooted in the base of your neck. Sitting up straight with your shoulders back and down can protect the nerve from irritation.
- **Lighten your bag.** Schlepping a handbag heavier than a toddler is a potential tension trigger.
- **Try some shower power.** When you feel stressed, a warm shower can help ease tense muscles.

It's probably a migraine if

- Your headaches tend to strike at the same time during your menstrual cycle each month.
- You get a headache after you consume red wine, aged cheese or the food additive MSG.
- You feel a throbbing pain on one side of the head, often with nausea or visual disturbances.

HEAD IT OFF
- **Keep a log.** Establish when the pain comes on and abates. Discuss the findings with your doctor.
- **Maintain a consistent sleep schedule.**
- **Eat a magnesium-rich diet.** The mineral affects levels of serotonin and other brain chemicals related to migraine. Whole grains, peanut butter, spinach and almonds are all good sources.

⏱ GOT 10 MINUTES? Manage migraines—naturally

Try out one of these drug-free pain fighters and enjoy relief.

GET NEEDLED Having acupuncture can prevent migraines as effectively as taking prescription drugs, a study in *The Lancet Neurology* shows. Find a licensed practitioner in your neighborhood at MedicalAcupuncture.org.

BELLY BREATHE Put one hand on your chest and one on your abdomen. Inhale and exhale slowly for 60 seconds while counting. You'll help curb muscle contraction and the release of hormones associated with migraines.

MAKE SMART FOOD CHOICES Cheese, chocolate, citrus fruit, cured meats and red wine contain natural chemicals that can trigger pain. To discover your personal food connections, log what you ate before pain began.

CONSIDER TAKING A SUPPLEMENT If you get three or more migraines a month, popping 200 milligrams of riboflavin or 75 mg of butterbur twice a day may cut occurrence in half. Ask your M.D. if one of them is right for you.

GOT 4 MINUTES?
Watch your back

AN ACHING BACK is the second most common reason (after colds) that people call in sick, according to the American Academy of Orthopedic Surgeons in Rosemont, Illinois. Stop the pain before it starts.

DURING HEAVY LIFTING Carry your load in front of you, against your abdomen. You get a mini-workout for your arms instead of a pain in the back.

AT YOUR DESK Hunching over your keyboard or crossing your legs can distribute your weight unevenly and place excessive pressure on your pelvis and gluteal muscles. Your weight should be centered over your sitz bones (the ones at the base of your butt). Keep your knees bent at a 90-degree angle by placing feet flat on the floor or on a footrest if necessary.

BEHIND THE WHEEL Driving, like any seated activity, increases pressure on the back. The stress is even greater while you're on the highway, most likely because of the vibrations. Without slouching, sit so your back is fully supported against the seat, which disperses some of the weight. If you can't sit this way comfortably after adjusting your seat, use a lumbar pad to bolster your lower back. During long trips, try to stop every 45 minutes or so to stand and stretch out.

WHILE YOU'RE WALKING Sure, you look sexy in your stilettos, but high heels shift your weight forward, forcing you to arch your back to maintain balance. After a mere couple of hours, the position can stress your back muscles and ligaments, says Michael R. Marks, M.D., president of the Connecticut Orthopedics Society in West Hartford. "If you can't give up high heels, at least minimize the time you're in them," Dr. Marks says, and save them for special occasions. Also, opt for thicker heels, which will give you better balance. Wearing flats with a cushioned, supportive sole is ideal.

GOT 30 SECONDS?

Fight wrist pain

Switch your mouse from one side of the computer to the other regularly to prevent wrist-tendon inflammation from the constant clicking.

GOT 3 MINUTES?
Release tense hips

Stretch your hips regularly. Sitting for long periods can stiffen them, causing back pain. Sit on the floor cross-legged and walk your hands as far forward as you can. Hold until you feel a release in your hips and lower back, then walk them back. Repeat, walking hands to each side. Switch legs and repeat entire sequence.

GOT 2 MINUTES?
Nix neck pain

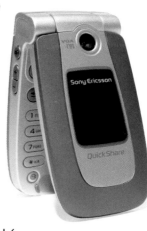

Between the computer hunch and the cellphone scrunch, your poor neck muscles take a beating. Consider wearing a headset to chat, and check that your computer monitor is at eye level (you may need to adjust your chair).

GOT 5 MINUTES?
Ease achy joints

The old saying is that cold hands signal a warm heart, but cool temps (indoors or out) actually take a toll on your joints. Soothe the stiffness with this hot-towel treatment: Fill a bowl with 3 cups hot water, ½ cup Epsom salts and 3 tablespoons witch hazel. Soak a terry towel in the mixture, wring it out and wrap your achy joints until the towel cools. The witch hazel helps the salt's minerals penetrate and relieve soreness.

⏱ GOT 15 MINUTES (OR LESS)?

Do a little "pre-hab" The two keys to defending against tenderness: building muscular endurance and correcting imbalances. Try these stretches regularly. You can even do them in the office or in front of the TV!

②ᴍɪɴ Leg lift Protects neck, back, wrists, knees Stand about 3 feet away from a sturdy desk or kitchen counter. With legs straight, heels planted, lean forward and place hands on desk, back slightly arched, arms straight. Bend right knee and slowly draw it into chest, moving from hip. Then, keeping knee bent, extend leg back, gently pressing sole of foot up toward ceiling. Do eight reps. Switch sides; repeat.

③ᴍɪɴ Wall sit plus Protects wrists, knees Squat with back to a wall, feet hip-width apart, thighs almost parallel to the floor. Maintain butt contact with wall as you lean torso forward slightly and raise arms, elbows bent 90 degrees. Remain in a squatting position while circling wrists 10 times in each direction. Stand up, rest 30 seconds and repeat entire sequence for one rep. Do four reps.

③ᴍɪɴ Figure-four stretch Protects back Sit on a chair with back straight, right ankle resting on left knee, left foot flat on floor. Grasp sides of chair with both hands as you slowly lean forward from hips, back flat. Hold for 30 seconds; switch sides for one rep. Do three reps.

①ᴍɪɴ Chest expansion
Protects neck, back
Stand with feet hip-width apart, arms at sides, hands in loose fists with thumbs out. Extend arms to shoulder height, thumbs facing each other. Bend elbows 90 degrees and point thumbs directly behind you while you move elbows out to the side. Return to start and repeat for one rep. Do five reps.

②ᴍɪɴ Side lean Protects neck, back, wrists, knees Stand with left side facing a sturdy desk or kitchen counter about 3 feet away. With legs together, lean to left and place left hand firmly on desk, right arm out to side at shoulder height, palm forward. Hold the position as you lift right leg toward ceiling, then lower it, for one rep. Do 10 reps. Switch sides and repeat.

①ᴍɪɴ Hinge and lift Protects neck, back, heels Stand with right foot at a comfortable distance in front of left, heels firmly planted and arms down. With legs straight, bend forward at hips, lowering chest to hip level, and reach forward. Keep arms extended as you return to upright position, then arch back slightly and return to start. Switch legs and repeat for one rep. Do five reps.

①ᴍɪɴ Shoulder spread Protects neck, back Stand with your back pressed against wall, feet together, arms out to sides at shoulder height, palms forward. Maintain contact with the wall as you slowly bend elbows to 90 degrees, pointing fingers toward ceiling. Straighten arms and repeat for one rep. Do three reps.

②ᴍɪɴ Reach and rock
Protects neck, back
Kneel on all fours, knees under hips, hands under shoulders and back flat. Keeping left hand planted and abs tight, rock hips forward and reach straight ahead with right arm. Hold for five seconds. Bring arm down; drop hips over heels and relax. Repeat on other side for one rep. Do five reps.

GOT 30 SECONDS?

Freeze that headache
Peas can help a pounding head. Use a 16-ounce bag of frozen ones to relieve your ache. It's cheap, and the bag molds perfectly to your forehead.

YOUR HEALTH TO-DON'T LIST

» Don't speed. For every 10 miles per hour over 50 mph you drive, the risk for death in an accident doubles.

» Don't pop a blister. Just let it be. It's the body's natural bandage.

» Don't slouch over a book. Reading in a supported horizontal position is much easier on your back than sitting.

» Don't overdo the mouthwash. Swishing with an alcohol-based rinse more than a few times a day can dry saliva, making your mouth's natural bacteria fighter less effective.

» Don't power through. Afternoon naps are actually good for you—not to mention absolutely delightful!

» Don't bother with air fresheners. A compound in many may reduce lung function. Use baking soda instead.

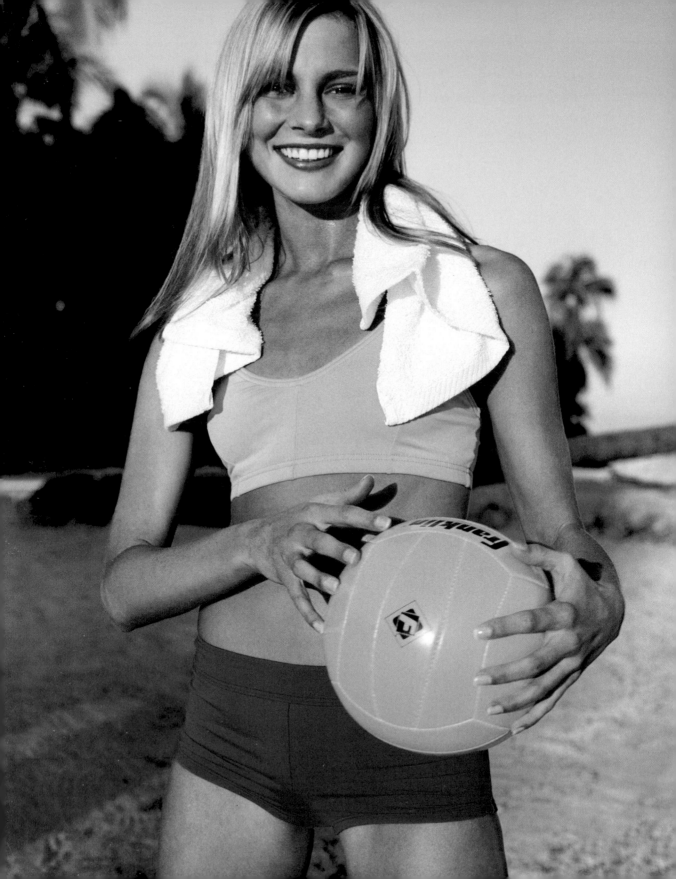

SHORTCUTS TO A
great body

Sneak in only a handful of these mini muscle-sculpting routines and lightning-quick calorie burners to look slimmer and sexier (and feel happier and healthier) in almost no time flat. Mojo a little low? No worries. You'll also find plenty of cinchy tricks to help make any workout—and we do mean *any* workout—feel even easier. Getting fit fast is about to become a lot more fun!

The only 10 things you need to know to achieve a sexy, strong and sleek physique

At SELF, we believe that getting in shape should be simple, fast, energizing and uplifting, not, repeat, *not* complicated, time-consuming, expensive or exhausting. If you have a pair of sneakers, a little motivation and a few minutes to spare, then you already have all it takes to achieve your strongest, sexiest, healthiest body ever. Use these get-fit guidelines to transform head to toe in a matter of weeks.

1 Just move it

You don't have to do anything fancy, like join a swanky gym, hire a trainer or buy a treadmill. Simply go for a walk. Clean your house. Dance. Be active 30 minutes a day most days of the week and you'll enjoy all of the amazing health perks exercise has to offer. You'll reduce your risk for heart disease, diabetes, many cancers, depression, osteoporosis and more. You'll also have more energy and less stress. And, oh, yeah, you'll score a smokin' body to boot. The best part: There's really no need to do it all at once. Breaking up your workout into two 15-minute sessions or three 10-minute bursts delivers the same good-for-you results, as long as you rev your heart rate during each effort.

2 If it hurts, stop

There's "my muscles are burning" pain, and then there's "I don't think my leg is supposed to bend that way" pain. The first kind? Perfectly normal. The second? That's a problem. If you ever feel that kind of ouch midmove, stop immediately. Or if you're super sore for more than a few days post-workout, check with your doctor to make sure everything is fine. (If it is, try the techniques on page 40 to prevent problems in the future.) Above all, trust your instincts; they're usually right.

3 Have fun

There is no golden rule that says working out must be grueling or unpleasant to bring you results. Quite the opposite, in fact. If you make exercise enjoyable, you'll actually be more likely to sweat a little longer and a little more often. Women who train in order to have fun, socialize, feel energized or be happier spend 40 percent more time exercising than women who work out simply to look good, a study from the University of Michigan at Ann Arbor found. So, what exercise suits you best? Imagine you had a day to do whatever activity sounded good. (No, a movie marathon doesn't count.) Would you garden? Play tag with your kids? Neither activity requires the old "no pain, no gain" school of thought, but both will strengthen your muscles, increase your heart rate and make you fitter and happier.

4 Ask for support

Exercise is more effective (and pleasurable) when you're with a friend. Research from Brown Medical School in Providence, Rhode Island, suggests that people trying to lose weight are likelier to stick with diet and exercise if they team up with someone who has already shed pounds. Plan a workout with a pal; whoever cancels buys dinner. Or enlist a buddy to keep you gung ho with phone reminders to hit the gym. Married? Co-opt your honey. Couples who work out together are less likely to quit exercising.

5 Don't overdo it

Going hog wild—working out too long, too hard or too often—is a surefire recipe for quick burnout and possibly injury. Take two days off a week to recover, and give your muscles 48 hours to rest and repair themselves between strength training sessions. (You can do cardio on interim days, if you'd like.)

6 Tone all over

Three quick reasons why you should get smart about dumbbells: (1) Weight training is the key to sculpting sexy muscles. You can melt all the fat you want, but if you've got nothing curvy underneath, you're only going to look like a mushy string bean. Choose a weight heavy enough so the last two reps feel tough to eke out. (2) Lifting weights helps keep your bones strong, lowering your risk for osteoporosis. If you do two strength sessions a week for a year, you'll increase your bone density by 1 percent—a huge improvement. (3) Your worries about looking like The Rock are unfounded. Women's physiology won't let us bulk up.

7 Get your heart pumping

If your ticker isn't beating faster than usual, then you need to work harder to reap all the great benefits of exercise. What's the right intensity? Either you can take your pulse and do some quick math to calculate your target heart rate (we show you how on page 254), or the easier option is the talk test. If you can sing along effortlessly with your MP3 player, you're exercising at low intensity; consider kicking it up a notch. If you can chat with your workout buddy but are too winded to sing, then you're moving at a moderate pace. Think of this as the Goldilocks pace: not too hard and not too easy, just right. If you can barely get two syllables out between breaths, your pace is very intense, which is hard to sustain. To build endurance, ease up a touch.

8 Warm up

Always front-end your workout with an easy 5 to 10 minutes of light cardio. Not only will it help prevent injury by improving muscle elasticity, but it will also assist you in burning more calories during the rest of your workout by jump-starting your metabolism.

9 Cool down

Post-exercise, take a few minutes to taper off. In a study at Springfield College in Massachusetts, exercisers who cooled down after a long, intense session perceived their workout to be less taxing and more pleasant than those who had easier or shorter workouts. Researchers hypothesize that the pleasing ending may be what you wind up associating with the workout, rather than the tougher get-sweaty part. Once you've brought down your heart rate, stretch. It will release muscle tension, reduce soreness and keep you lithe and agile.

10 Mix it up

Even if you love your workout, you need to make changes every few weeks. The longer you stick with a program, the more efficient your body becomes at doing it. You end up using less energy and burning fewer calories, and you won't get optimal results. That doesn't mean you have to ditch your favorite routine altogether. Even small tweaks (find loads of 'em in this chapter) should help you make progress. Up your intensity, vary your sets and reps, use different weights, swap in new moves or flip the order of your current ones. Such switches will keep your body challenged—and keep your mind engaged, too.

⏱ GOT 3 MINUTES? Help exercise seem easier

Try these sneaky mind games to feel bionic—or at least a little more bouncy—the next time your workout needs some juice.

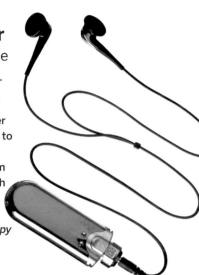

TALK BACK

Replace those downer thoughts like "I'll never last 20 minutes on a run" with a happy-place word like *beach* or a mantra such as "I'm invincible!" for a midsession lift, Joseph Rembisz, a hypnotherapist in New York City, advises.

RESET YOUR BRAIN

Flutter your eyelashes for three seconds, then blink slowly three times. The fast switch between light and dark triggers a mind-refresh reflex for a psychological surge, says Kay Porter, Ph.D., a sports psychologist in Eugene, Oregon.

BUILD A PLAYLIST

Pick an MP3 player over the TV as a gym buddy to feel more positive as you sweat, a study from Elon University in North Carolina suggests. Other research in the *Journal of Music Therapy* found tunes can also help you walk farther.

⏱ GOT 15 MINUTES?
Wake up gym-ready

Even if you're not a morning person, A.M. workouts make sense: In a study of fitness-class goers at the Southwest Health Institute in Phoenix, 75 percent of those who exercised first thing stuck with the program as opposed to those who waited until lunch (50 percent) or after work (35 percent). To join the rise-and-sweat crowd, wake up 15 minutes earlier one week, a half hour earlier the next and so on, until there's time to do your routine. Obey your new alarm for two more weeks to ingrain the schedule and feel newly energetic!

⏱ GOT 5 MINUTES?
Kick-start your routine

SO YOU SWORE to get moving? Up your chances for success:

☐ **TAKE A PLEDGE** In a study at Washington State University at Pullman, gymgoers who were asked in a mailing, "Will you work out?" were more likely to do so than those whose mailer didn't include the question. "Consciously committing to exercise could increase your odds of going to the gym from 37 to 63 percent," says study author David Sprott, Ph.D. Jot down your mission statement on a separate piece of paper and post it on your medicine cabinet or night table, where you'll see it often.

☐ **MAKE A DATE** Pencil in a workout on your calendar on every Monday for the next month. "Exercising the first day of the workweek sets a psychological pattern, so you'll be more likely to do your routine each day that follows," says Wayne Westcott, Ph.D., fitness research director at the South Shore YMCA in Quincy, Massachusetts. Plus, writing it down can make you more accountable.

☐ **CLOCK YOUR MINUTES** Set a time limit for your workout beforehand—it may make each stride or repetition seem more manageable. Joggers at the University of Cape Town in South Africa who were told to run for 20 minutes found a treadmill session easier than runners who didn't know how long they had to go. Knowledge really is power!

◷ GOT 5 MINUTES?

Motivate yourself to move

There are times when you just can't seem to get your body—or mind—in gear to exercise. SELF rounded up the science behind the biggest motivation busters and boosters to help you get going. Learn and lace up!

Top 5 motivation busters

1 **THERE'S NO TIME** Instead of hemming and hawing, simply go to the gym. A study from the University of Alberta in Edmonton found it's key for women to simply start moving instead of overthinking.

2 **NOBODY'S CHEERING** Studies show people with support exercise more regularly. Make a standing date with a buddy to help yourself stay on track.

3 **MY HOUSE IS TOO COMFY** You don't have to leave it! A study in the *Journal of the American Medical Association* showed home cardio-machine users were more likely to keep at it than people sans equipment. No machine? Pop in a workout DVD.

4 **MY BODY NEVER CHANGES** To break through a plateau, switch up your routine. Exercisers who alternated moderate- and high-intensity cardio intervals burned nine times more fat than the moderate-only group in a study at Laval University in Quebec. When you're toning, change the reps and weight between strength sessions.

5 **IT'S TOO PRICEY** A gym can be costly until you consider that non-exercisers average at least $330 more yearly in medical bills than active people. Ask your boss to subsidize fees. (More than a third of employers do so.)

Top 5 motivation boosters

1 **DO IT FOR YOU** "The more you exercise to please others or assuage guilt, the less likely you'll be to stick with it," says Wendy Rodgers, Ph.D., exercise psychologist at the University of Alberta in Edmonton.

2 **HAVE A GOAL** "Set a target that is specific, actionable, short-term and measurable," suggests James Annesi, Ph.D., wellness director at the YMCA of Metropolitan Atlanta. Fine-tune "I want to lose weight" to "I want to fit into a size 10 in six weeks."

3 **FOLLOW A PROGRAM** If you have a plan before you exercise—find loads of monthly programs at Self.com—"then you're accountable to it, and you'll feel more satisfied once you fulfill it," says Tom Holland, an exercise physiologist in Darien, Connecticut. And the better you feel, the more likely you'll exercise again.

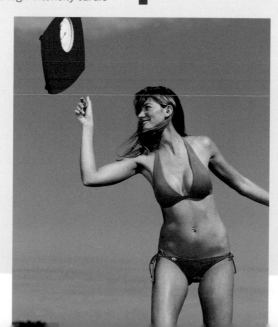

4 **IGNORE THE SCALE** Research suggests that post-exercise, you'll feel slimmer before the digits back you up. "You'll benefit from an improved mood and a sense of mastery, promoting better body image," Annesi says. Let those good vibes buoy you until the scale budges.

5 **SENSE SUCCESS** Imagine a great workout and it can happen. Visualizing it a few minutes a day can alter behavior, science shows.

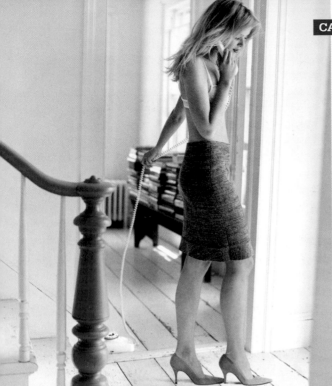

GOT 2 MINUTES?
Set a slim-down goal to incinerate 300 calories

To shed fat fast, here's the minimum number of minutes of your favorite cardio to do per exercise session.

Activity	»	Minutes*
Inline skating	»	22
Jumping rope	»	28
Running (6 mph)	»	28
Stair climbing	»	31
Jogging (5 mph)	»	35
Bicycling (13 mph)	»	35
Aerobics (high intensity)	»	40
Dancing (aerobic)	»	43
Elliptical (moderate pace)	»	43
Hiking	»	47
Swimming	»	47
Aerobics (low intensity)	»	56
Walking (4 mph)	»	56

*All times are based on a 135-pound woman.

GOT 1 MINUTE?
Get on your feet

Offer your seat on the bus or stand up when you answer the phone—it may mean a fitter you. Even when you're doing absolutely nothing, standing burns 17 percent more calories than sitting. Going vertical may make a difference of up to 350 calories a day (which equals 3 pounds per month), researchers at the Mayo Clinic in Rochester, Minnesota, report. Overweight people in the study spent about two and a half more hours daily in their chair than did their lean colleagues.

GOT 1 MINUTE?
Give yourself a cardio checkup Take this quiz
to see if you should rev your sweat sessions or lay off a little bit.

4 signs you're slacking off
☐ You chat on the phone during exercise.
☐ You often sport the same gym clothes two days in a row. Why not? They don't stink!
☐ You've been walking/jogging/cycling for a good hour and haven't even broken a sweat.
☐ You've stopped seeing any better-body results.

4 signs you're overdoing it
☐ You're having a hard time sleeping.
☐ Your appetite is gone despite tough workouts.
☐ You are suffering from stress fractures or chronic muscle soreness or have stopped menstruating.
☐ Your honey actually suggests taking separate vacations because you're so darn cranky.

⊕ GOT 1 MINUTE? Know the magic numbers of weight loss

Shedding pounds is simple math. Abide by this cheat sheet and watch the scale do some subtraction.

3,500 = Expend this many total calories weekly above the amount that you take in to lose 1 pound.

300 = Burn this number of calories per session to be in the weight loss zone. (See how in box at left.)

250 = Spend at least this many minutes exercising each week to be on the fast track to Slimville.

2 = Drop no more than this many pounds per week to ensure you're losing weight at a sustainable rate.

⊕ GOT 3 MINUTES?
Play to lose (fat, that is)

TRY THESE tweaks to your routine to maximize fat melting.

DIVIDE IT UP Slice and dice cardio for a better postworkout fat burn, scientists from the University of Tokyo suggest. Exercisers who did two half-hour stints of moderate cycling with a 20-minute rest in between burned 10 percent more fat afterward than when they cycled straight for one hour. The repeated bouts triggered a release of hormones that helped metabolize fat more efficiently so that fat supplied a greater percentage of the total calories used later.

DO INTERVALS Alternating your pace or intensity within one workout spurs fat loss. Women who spent 20 minutes mixing sprints with jogging lost three times the fat off their legs and butt in 15 weeks as those jogging steadily for 40 minutes, a study from the University of New South Wales in Sydney finds.

LIFT FIRST If you tone and do cardio in the same session, you may want to start with weights. In another study from the University of Tokyo, exercisers who did a total-body strength workout 20 minutes before cycling burned 10 percent more fat than those who simply cycled. Lifting also taps those hormones that guide fat into the furnace. The reverse (doing cardio, then weights) doesn't.

⊕ GOT 1 MINUTE?
Ace a pace

Speed bursts are the secret to fast-tracking fat burn, but how quickly should you aim to go? Find your age and your top speed (recommended by health experts) below. Then push yourself to hit it when doing intervals.

How fast should you be able to run?	
AGE	TOP SPEED
20	6.1 to 7.2 mph
25	5.7 to 6.8 mph
30	5.4 to 6.4 mph
35	5.0 to 6.0 mph
40	4.6 to 5.6 mph
45	4.2 to 5.2 mph

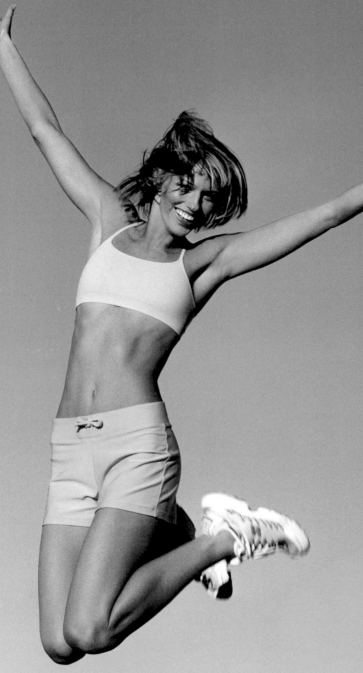

GOT 10 MINUTES?

Burn more calories!

THE GOAL Fight flab and sculpt your body from head to toe with this 10-minute workout made of the best fat burners from SELF's Body Bonus routines. These exercises are fast-paced and full-body to maximize the sizzle!

THE PLAN Perform these moves three times a week as a circuit, with only enough rest in between to hydrate if necessary. Repeat the series if you can. No equipment needed! Do the routine for four weeks for a sleek body.

THE PAYOFF You can't help but get leaner all over.

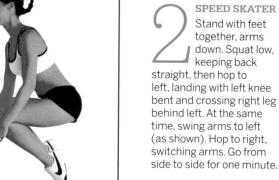

1 HOP TUCK

Stand with feet hip-width apart, knees soft, arms raised to shoulder level, palms down. Squat until knees are bent about 90 degrees. Jump up, bringing knees toward chest as you grab them with both hands (as shown). Land in squat; repeat for 30 seconds.

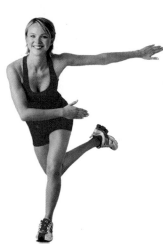

2 SPEED SKATER

Stand with feet together, arms down. Squat low, keeping back straight, then hop to left, landing with left knee bent and crossing right leg behind left. At the same time, swing arms to left (as shown). Hop to right, switching arms. Go from side to side for one minute.

3 STAR JUMPER

Stand with feet hip-width apart, arms down. Inhale as you squat, keeping heels on floor and chest high; touch floor with hands. Exhale and leap up, arms and legs wide, reaching toward ceiling (as shown). Land softly with knees bent and squat again right away. Do five jumps, then rest for 10 breaths. Repeat twice.

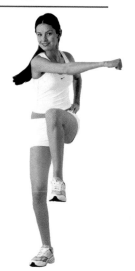

4 CROSS PUNCH

March in place quickly to start, swinging arms and raising knees as high as possible. After one minute, slow the pace and raise left knee as you contract abs and punch right arm across body until right elbow is in line with knee (as shown). Switch arms and legs. Continue alternating for two minutes.

5 MOUNTAIN CLIMBER

Get into push-up position on hands and toes. Keeping hips low and head in line with spine, alternate bringing one knee at a time toward chest (as shown). When you get a feel for the move, increase the pace and switch legs in midair, keeping toes off floor. Repeat for one minute.

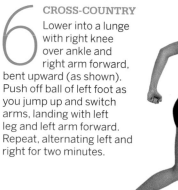

6 CROSS-COUNTRY

Lower into a lunge with right knee over ankle and right arm forward, bent upward (as shown). Push off ball of left foot as you jump up and switch arms, landing with left leg and left arm forward. Repeat, alternating left and right for two minutes.

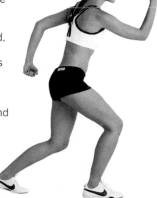

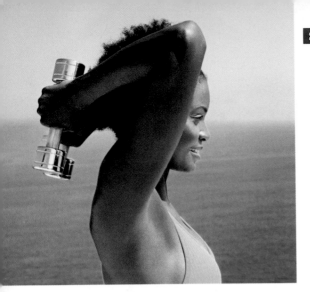

⏱ GOT 4 MINUTES?
Learn how to sculpt wisely

So you've hit a rut with your dumbbells. Find the firming fix for whatever is subverting your sculpting results.

PROBLEM "It's taking forever to get in shape."
SOLUTION Vary reps and weights between strength sessions. For example: Monday, do 12 to 15 lightweight reps per move; Wednesday, 3 to 5 heavy reps; Friday, 8 to 10 moderate reps. Repeat. Women in a study in *Medicine & Science in Sport & Exercise* got stronger this way than by sticking to 8 to 12 reps each session.

PROBLEM "I have some definition but want more."
SOLUTION Pick weights that fatigue your muscles within 15 repetitions. If you can easily do more reps than that with the weight you're using, it isn't heavy enough to add definition, says physiologist Ron Cox, Ph.D., at Miami University in Oxford, Ohio.

PROBLEM "I'm short on time most days."
SOLUTION Do reps in one second up, one second down. A study at the University of Sydney discovered that exercisers who sped up the reps gained 11 percent more strength in one set than those who did lifts of six seconds.

PROBLEM "I'm scared to bulk up."
SOLUTION Lift! Women don't have enough muscle-building testosterone to get bulky, even using heavy weights. "Some will gain muscle faster than they lose fat, so they may be bigger until they shed some of the flab, " says Tom Seabourne, Ph.D., director of exercise science at Northeast Texas Community College in Mount Pleasant.

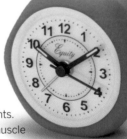

⏱ GOT 3 MINUTES?
Discover the way to train for better bones

TURNS OUT, calcium alone may not be enough for strong bones. In a study from California State Polytechnic University at Pomona, sedentary women ages 20 to 35 did not increase bone density despite hitting the RDA of the mineral. Get your calcium, *and* try these strengtheners.

UPPER BODY Lat pull-downs, rowing moves, overhead presses, back extension machine: Three sets of 8 to 10 reps each, twice a week, raised overall density by 2 percent in six months.

HIPS Squats and the leg-press machine (three sets of 8 to 10 reps each, twice a week) improved hip density by 1.6 percent in six months.

LEGS Weight-bearing cardio such as aerobics, jumping rope or jogging is also key. Women who did Step classes three times a week saw leg bone density rise about 1 percent in six months.

✳ ⏱GOT 10 MINUTES? Firm your tummy at the office

"Inch your body away from the chair back and straighten up for 10 minutes each hour," says Debra Strougo, a trainer in New York City. "Imagine there's wet paint on the seat back." Now that's middle management!

🕐 GOT 15 MINUTES?

Sneak in some toning

You can transform all those little daily tasks into quickie strength exercise sessions. Check out the chart below to see how you can earn credit for fitness minutes throughout the day. Aiming for 15 is a good start.

2 MINUTES
- Do 50 heel raises while waiting in line.
- Squeeze glutes 50 times as you brush.
- Sneak in 50 crunches during commercials.

5 MINUTES
- Got stairs? Climb eight flights daily.
- Do 50 deep pliés while making phone calls.
- Carry 12 bags of groceries from the car.

10 MINUTES
- Sweep and mop your kitchen floor.
- Fold and put away the week's laundry.
- Fill and carry a cartload of groceries.

15 MINUTES
- Mow the lawn or prune the hedge.
- Shovel a snowy driveway—bend at knees!
- Wash and dry your car in loving detail.

🕐 GOT 1 MINUTE?

Strive for balance

Balance training improves muscle coordination, which means better firming, suggest researchers at the University of Rostock in Germany. Stand one-legged on a folded towel while doing biceps curls for muscle-priming perks. Or use a Wobble Board—a mini-seesaw for feet—at the gym for one-minute bouts.

🕐 GOT 10 MINUTES?

Get great gams

Instead of avoiding stairs during your jog, tackle them two at a time. "When you skip every other step, you have to push off harder than when using a normal running stride," explains exercise physiologist Tom Holland. (To strengthen knees, concentrate on using your top leg to leverage your body weight up.) In 10 minutes, you'll burn 146 calories and force your body to overcome gravity by recruiting more muscle fibers. The payoff: a firm, sexy butt and great-looking legs you'll love.

GOT 30 SECONDS?

Give yourself a lift
Do a quick psych-up before your reps. In a study, women who visualized a newly toned self could hoist more weight than those who were distracted.

GOT 15 MINUTES?

Get fab abs

THE GOAL Create a flat, sexy midsection with our favorite foolproof firmers. See more ab moves at Self.com.

THE PLAN Work three or four of these exercises into your regimen three times a week. (Easing them in will minimize soreness.) After two weeks, try the entire routine during one session. Do the number of reps indicated, resting one minute between moves. The only equipment you'll need is a hand towel.

THE PAYOFF Extra room in your waistband within as little as one month

1 PIKE 90

Lie faceup; raise legs until perpendicular to floor, feet flexed. Lower right leg so it hovers 1 or 2 inches off floor and place hands lightly behind head. In this position, do 15 crunches, lifting chest toward ceiling and lowering (as shown). Switch legs and repeat.

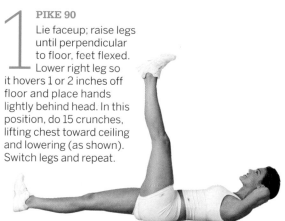

2 SLIDING CRUNCH

On a slippery floor, kneel on all fours, feet hip-width apart on a towel. Lift knees and inhale as you slide feet back until body is in a straight line, hands under shoulders. Slowly draw knees toward arms (as shown) on the exhale. Slide feet out, inhaling, until legs are straight again. Do 15 reps.

3 CRUNCHY FROG

Sit with knees bent, feet flat. Keeping legs together, raise feet several inches and bring knees toward chest. Wrap arms around knees without touching legs. Extend legs and stretch arms to sides, palms forward (as shown). Return to wrapped-arm position; repeat. Do 15 reps.

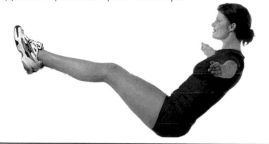

4 TORNADO

Stand with feet hip-width apart, right leg in front of left, right foot turned out. Bend elbows and raise arms out to sides at shoulder level (like goalposts). In one motion, raise right knee to lowered right elbow (as shown). Return to start; switch sides and repeat to complete one rep. Do 15 reps.

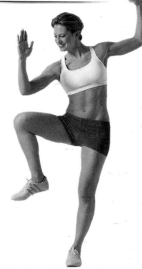

5 CORKSCREW

Lie faceup. Press legs together and raise them toward ceiling until they're at a 90-degree angle, with knees slightly bent and toes pointed. Raise butt and legs off floor using ab muscles; twist legs slightly to left (as shown). Repeat, twisting to right, for one rep. Do 15 reps.

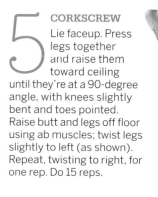

6 SIDE ARM BALANCE

Start on floor on knees. Lean to left and place left hand on floor under shoulder; extend right arm up and to left, palm down. Beginners, straighten right leg out to right with foot on floor, resting on left knee. For a challenge, extend both legs to right, knees off floor (as shown). Hold for 5 breaths. Return to start; switch sides. Repeat twice per side.

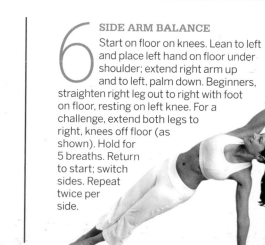

◷ GOT 1 MINUTE?
Tape this chart to your treadmill

To scorch 168 to 328 calories, walk or run through this half-hour treadmill plan from Burn 60 gym in Los Angeles three times a week.

Minutes	Phase	Walk	Run
2	Warm-up	3 mph	5 mph
2	Start	3.8 mph	5.8 mph
1	Sprint	4.2 mph	6.5 mph
2	Recovery	3 mph	5.5 mph
1	Sprint	4.3 mph	6.8 mph
2	Recovery	3 mph	5.5 mph
1	Sprint	4.4 mph	7 mph
2	Recovery	3.5 mph	6 mph
1	Sprint	4.4 mph	7.5 mph
2	Recovery	3.5 mph	5.5 mph
1	Sprint	4.6 mph	8 mph
2	Recovery	4 mph	6.5 mph
1	Sprint	4.8 mph	8.5 mph
2	Recovery	4 mph	6.5 mph
2	Hill intervals	4 mph Incline 2%	6.5 mph Incline 2%
1	Recovery	4 mph Incline 0.5 %	6.5 mph Incline 0.5%
2	Hill intervals	4.5 mph Incline 4%	6.5 mph Incline 4%
1	Recovery	4.5 mph Incline 0.5%	6.5 mph Incline 0.5%
2	Cooldown	3 mph	5 mph

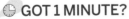

◷ GOT 1 MINUTE?
Make your walk sizzle

"At a 12- or 13-minute-mile pace, you naturally want to jog because it's physically easier; it takes less energy than it does to walk," says Therese Ikonian, author of *Walking Fast* (Human Kinetics). Squelch the urge—you'll use more calories; 20 minutes of a 5 mph walk burns 172 calories versus 150 for a 5 mph jog.

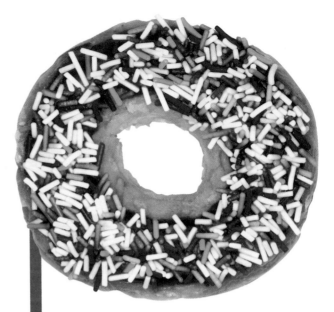

◷ GOT 3 MINUTES?
Feel inspired to hoof it

FOR THOSE LOW on motivation to move, walking is the easiest entrée to exercise. Need an extra push to try it? Consider how a stroll can combat...

JUNK FOOD Eating fatty foods (hello, doughnuts!) can cause arteries to lose elasticity for six hours, but exercise can buffer the effect, scientists at Indiana University at Bloomington suggest. Study participants who walked for 45 minutes two hours after a fast food breakfast maintained the same healthy heart function as those who ate a fat-free meal and then rested. Stride to deactivate that fat bomb.

ANXIETY For a calmer head, take a brisk stroll. People on the verge of a panic attack who walked 30 minutes were twice as likely to dodge the episode as those who rested quietly, a study from Charité University Hospital in Berlin reports. Step out as soon as you feel you're nearing the breaking point, as anxiety can escalate in only 5 to 10 minutes.

THE BLUES No doubt exercise can work as a happy pill, but what's the right dose? You see peak mood benefits by walking 11 to 19 miles a week (only 2 miles a day!), a study at the University of Texas Southwestern Medical Center in Dallas finds.

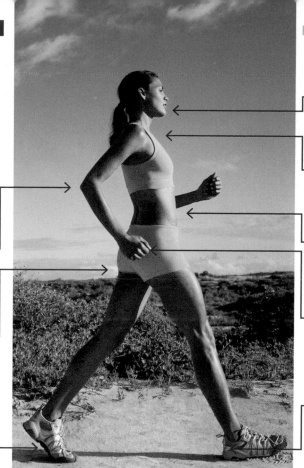

⏱ GOT 2 MINUTES?
Perfect your form
Get the most out of every stride today.

Chin
Look forward, not down, so chin stays parallel to ground.

Shoulders
Drop shoulders down and back to ensure better posture.

Abs
Pull abs in tight to keep torso tall and chest lifted.

Arms
Swing arms from front to back for extra help propelling yourself forward.

Heel
Land on heel of forward leg with knee slightly bent. Keep knees soft as you go.

Elbows
Keep elbows bent at about a 90-degree angle. Imagine you're marching.

Butt
Squeeze glutes as you push off rear foot; it will tone your tush with each step.

Forefoot
Press off from ball of rear foot to derive added leverage and spring.

⏱ GOT 5 MINUTES? Map out your "I want to run" goal
If you're a walker—or a walk-jogger—follow this quickie guide to running a 5K.

WEEK 1	WEEK 2	WEEK 3	WEEK 4
WORKOUT 1 Warm up for a few minutes, then jog easily for two minutes. Slow down and walk fast for a minute. Repeat jog-walk sequence six times.	**WORKOUT 1** Warm up for a few minutes, then jog easily for four minutes. Walk fast for a minute. Repeat jog-walk sequence three times.	**WORKOUT 1** Warm up for two minutes. Jog easily for eight minutes, then walk fast for one. Repeat sequence twice for a total of 24 minutes of jogging.	**WORKOUT 1** Warm up for two minutes, then run for 30 minutes at a moderate pace (you can talk). Be sure to walk for five minutes to cool down.
WORKOUT 2 Repeat workout 1, but jog for three minutes at a time instead of two. Repeat jog-walk sets five times.	**WORKOUT 2** Repeat workout 1, but jog for six minutes at a time instead of four. Repeat jog-walk sequence twice.	**WORKOUT 2** Warm up for two minutes. Jog for 10 minutes, then walk fast 1 minute. Repeat jog-walk sequence twice.	**WORKOUT 2** Warm up for two minutes, then run for 35 minutes at an easy pace. Cool down for another five minutes.
WORKOUT 3 Take a break from running to do other cardio (swimming, biking, dancing) for 30 minutes.	**WORKOUT 3** Do your favorite cardio (besides running) for 30 minutes at moderate intensity.	**WORKOUT 3** As usual, it's your choice of cardio. This time, keep it up for 35 minutes. You can do it!	**WORKOUT 3** Warm up for 2 minutes; run for 40 minutes at an easy pace. Cool down five minutes.

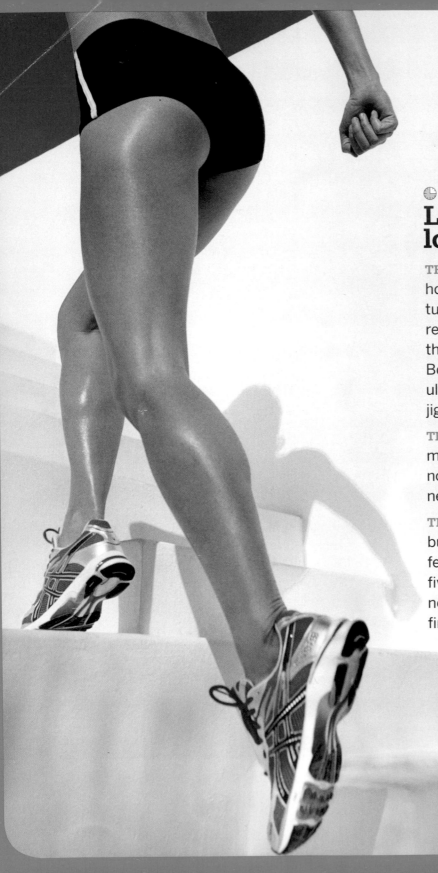

🕐 GOT 15 MINUTES?

Love your lower half

THE GOAL Achieve toned, honed hot legs and a tight tush with our lower-body reshaping plan, made of the best firmers from SELF's Body Bonus routines. This ultra-speedy regimen fights jiggle in a flash.

THE PLAN Do one set of each move three times a week on nonconsecutive days. All you need is a towel.

THE PAYOFF Your thighs and butt will appear tighter in as few as 10 days (that's about five workouts), and you'll notice short-shorts-worthy firming in only one month.

1 TOE-ROLL LUNGE

Assume a lunge position with right leg in front, knee over ankle, left leg extended straight back. Place hands on waist. Push off ball of left foot, rolling forward onto left toes (as shown), then back to heel, in one motion. Don't let front knee go past toes. Do 15 reps. Switch legs; repeat.

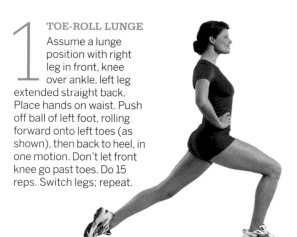

2 TIPTOE PLIÉ

Stand with heels together, toes out, arms in front at chest height with elbows bent, palms facing body. With heels touching, bend knees, rise onto balls of feet and lower as far as you can (as shown). Slowly straighten legs and repeat, without letting heels touch floor. Do 15 reps.

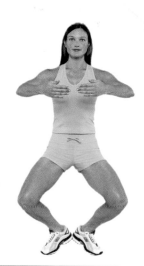

3 TOWEL SQUAT

Stand with left foot on a rolled towel (on a mat or carpet to prevent slipping), hands on hips. Raise right foot several inches in front of you, knee slightly bent. Keeping torso tall and chest raised, lower into a squat, bending left knee (as shown). Stand up. Do 15 reps. Switch legs; repeat.

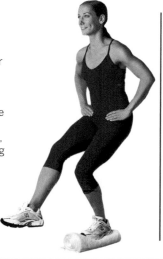

4 THREE-WAY KICK

Stand with feet hip-width apart, knees slightly bent, hands near face, elbows bent. With left leg, kick flexed foot to front, then to left (as shown) and back, tapping floor between kicks, for one rep. For balance, lean away, looking in direction of kick. Do 15 reps. Switch legs; repeat.

5 SKIER SQUAT WITH TWIST

Stand with feet together and lower into a squat. Bring palms together in prayer position and twist torso to right, placing back of left arm against outside of right leg and pointing right elbow toward ceiling. Look up to right (as shown). Hold for three counts. Stand and twist to left. Do 15 twists on each side.

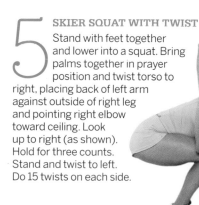

6 HOT SEAT

Stand with feet wide, toes turned out. Lower into a squat and hold shins, keeping head high. Hold one count, then, maintaining squat, release hands and lift torso. Extend arms out to sides at shoulder height, elbows bent 90 degrees, and contract biceps (as shown). Hold 15 counts, then stand up. Rest eight counts; repeat.

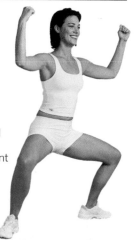

◔ GOT 3 MINUTES? Find your yoga style

Ever feel as if everyone else is blissfully at ease in yoga class while you're cowering self-consciously on your mat in a corner? Put an end to anxiety with this primer on choosing the class that best fits you, created with help from Jill Satterfield, founder of Vajra Yoga studio in New York City. Whether you're looking to sculpt or seek enlightenment, your first step—or pose—is to start here.

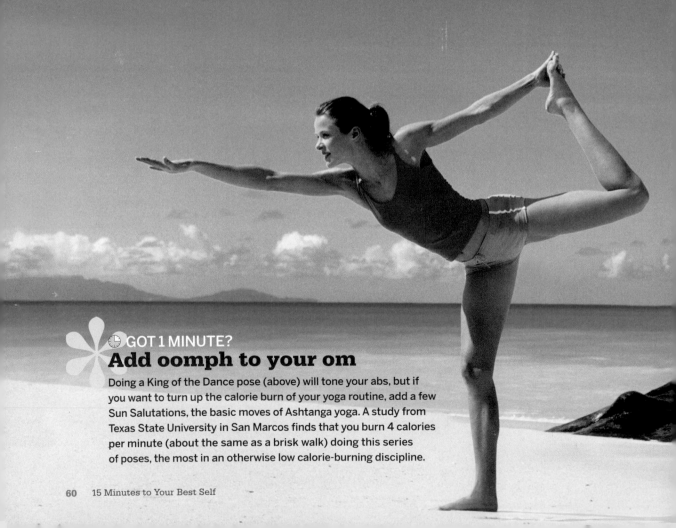

◔ GOT 1 MINUTE?
Add oomph to your om

Doing a King of the Dance pose (above) will tone your abs, but if you want to turn up the calorie burn of your yoga routine, add a few Sun Salutations, the basic moves of Ashtanga yoga. A study from Texas State University in San Marcos finds that you burn 4 calories per minute (about the same as a brisk walk) doing this series of poses, the most in an otherwise low calorie-burning discipline.

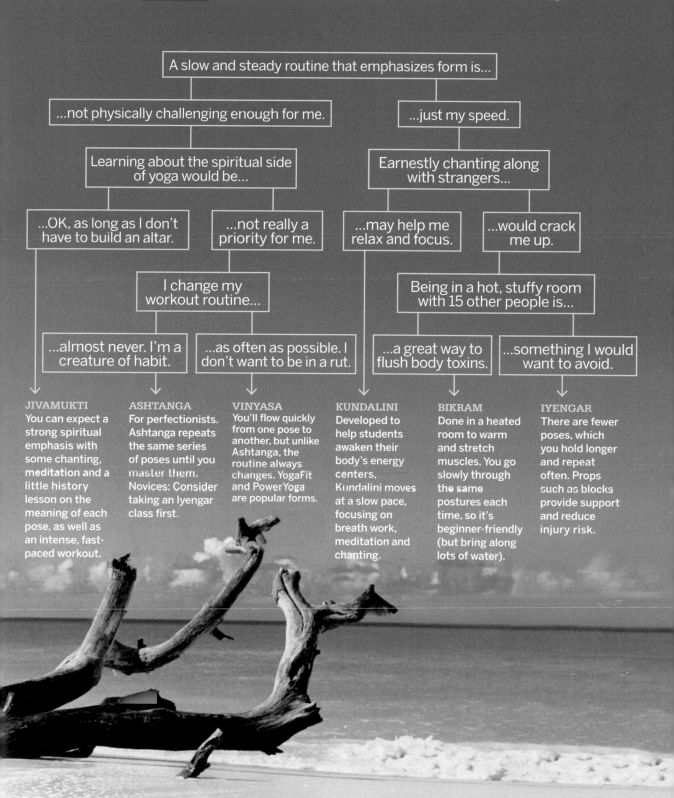

A slow and steady routine that emphasizes form is...

...not physically challenging enough for me.

...just my speed.

Learning about the spiritual side of yoga would be...

Earnestly chanting along with strangers...

...OK, as long as I don't have to build an altar.

...not really a priority for me.

...may help me relax and focus.

...would crack me up.

I change my workout routine...

Being in a hot, stuffy room with 15 other people is...

...almost never. I'm a creature of habit.

...as often as possible. I don't want to be in a rut.

...a great way to flush body toxins.

...something I would want to avoid.

JIVAMUKTI
You can expect a strong spiritual emphasis with some chanting, meditation and a little history lesson on the meaning of each pose, as well as an intense, fast-paced workout.

ASHTANGA
For perfectionists. Ashtanga repeats the same series of poses until you master them. Novices: Consider taking an Iyengar class first.

VINYASA
You'll flow quickly from one pose to another, but unlike Ashtanga, the routine always changes. YogaFit and PowerYoga are popular forms.

KUNDALINI
Developed to help students awaken their body's energy centers, Kundalini moves at a slow pace, focusing on breath work, meditation and chanting.

BIKRAM
Done in a heated room to warm and stretch muscles. You go slowly through the same postures each time, so it's beginner-friendly (but bring along lots of water).

IYENGAR
There are fewer poses, which you hold longer and repeat often. Props such as blocks provide support and reduce injury risk.

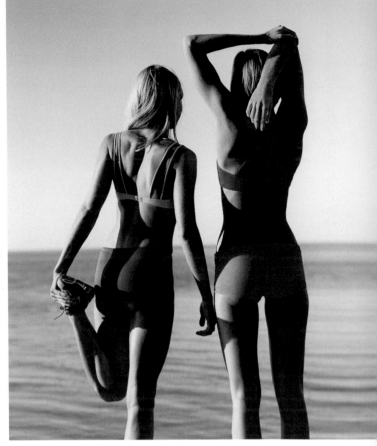

⊕ GOT 10 MINUTES?
Sweat smarter

SELF went to the foremost exercise experts to expose 10 popular fitness myths. Learn the real keys to getting results.

Myth 1 Muscle turns to fat.

THE TRUTH "Muscle and fat are two completely different tissues that have different functions," says Walter R. Thompson, Ph.D., professor of kinesiology, health and nutrition at Georgia State University in Atlanta. "One can't turn into the other." When you stop exercising, muscles atrophy, so you'll lose the tone you worked to attain. And if you overindulge at meals, you will gain fat.

Myth 2 You need to exercise 30 minutes straight to get fit.

THE TRUTH "Anything you do, for any period of time, will give you some benefit," says exercise scientist Matt Feigenbaum, Ph.D., at Furman University in Greenville, South Carolina. Plus, "You can accrue the same health benefits with three 10-minute bouts of aerobic exercise as during a 30-minute one." To lose weight, though, obviously the more you do, the faster you'll succeed.

Myth 3 Women naturally tend to lose extra weight from the top down.

THE TRUTH You may feel as if your breasts bear the brunt of your weight loss, but—good news for you tape measurers!—your belly generally takes the first hit. "Abdominal fat is more hormone- and enzyme-sensitive than fat in other areas, so your body may turn to it first when there's an energy deficiency," says Tom Seabourne, Ph.D., director of exercise science at Northeast Texas Community College. "The fat stored in the hips and thighs was designed to hang around in case of times of starvation, so it takes longer to get rid of."

Myth 4 Stretching before exercise will prevent injury and help performance.

THE TRUTH Researchers haven't yet shown conclusively that preworkout stretching cuts injury risk or improves performance. Limbering up can make bending, reaching, twisting and lifting easier, however, says Michael Bracko, Ed.D., a sports physiologist in Calgary, Alberta. Save stretching for post-exercise, when muscles are warm.

Myth 5 Overweight people typically have a sluggish metabolism.

THE TRUTH "Fewer than 10 percent of overweight people have metabolic disorders," says Jeffrey A. Potteiger, Ph.D., chair of the department of physical education, health and sport studies at Miami University in Oxford, Ohio. "The heavier you are, the more calories you burn during exercise at the same relative workload as a slimmer person." Gaining weight? Scrutinize your activity level.

Myth 6 You don't sweat as you swim.

THE TRUTH "If you're exerting yourself in the water, you will sweat," says Jane Katz, Ed.D., author of *Swimming for Total Fitness* (Broadway Books). "You just don't feel it because you're wet already." As with any exercise, be sure to sip a little H_2O before, during and after your workout. Bonus: Swimming burns 450 to 700 calories per hour!

Myth 7 You can target your upper and lower abdominal muscles separately.

THE TRUTH The rectus abdominis, or six-pack muscle that runs from your sternum to your pubic bone, is one muscle. "You can't work one end without the other," Seabourne says, although you might feel as if you are.

Myth 8 Pilates lengthens muscles.

THE TRUTH "The length of your muscles is predetermined and remains constant," says Michele S. Olson, Ph.D., professor of exercise science at Auburn University Montgomery in Alabama. Pilates can, however, improve flexibility and posture, which can make you *look* taller.

Myth 9 The calorie readout on cardio machines at the gym is accurate.

THE TRUTH Don't count on it, says John Porcari, Ph.D., professor of exercise science at the University of Wisconsin at La Crosse: "I've done studies on some of the newer types of machines that were as much as 70 percent off." The reason? Machines such as ellipticals haven't been around long enough for experts to develop the appropriate calorie-burn equations. Meanwhile, old-timers like bikes and treadmills are fairly precise.

Myth 10 To help you lose the most flab, exercise in the fat-burning zone.

THE TRUTH "Focus on total caloric expenditure, not where those calories are coming from," Thompson says. "If you want to burn 100 calories, it doesn't matter if you do it at 60 percent of your max heart rate [aka the fat-burning zone] or 85 percent. But the person working at 85 percent gets it done faster." Plus, you don't use adipose fat (flab) at low-intensity (60 to 70 percent of max); your body burns fatty acids and fat in the bloodstream.

⏱ GOT 6 MINUTES?
Test your fitness IQ Match the exercise to its health benefits and calories burned per half hour to see how your tried-and-true routine stacks up.

Body benefits	Calories	Exercise
1 This activity firms legs and strengthens heart and lungs, but you still need to tone your upper body.	209	Elliptical trainer
2 For every few hours of this activity you log weekly, you reduce your heart disease risk by 30 percent.	161	Running
3 Rest no more than 30 seconds between moves and this becomes a remarkably good cardio workout.	322	Walking (brisk)
4 Tone muscles with this stretch-and-strengthen regimen that weight machines often skip.	256	Yoga
5 This activity is as effective a calorie burner as walking at 4.5 miles per hour on a treadmill.	216	Circuit training

Answers 1 (322) **Running 2** (161) **Walking 3** (256) **Circuit training 4** (216) **Yoga 5** (209) **Elliptical trainer**

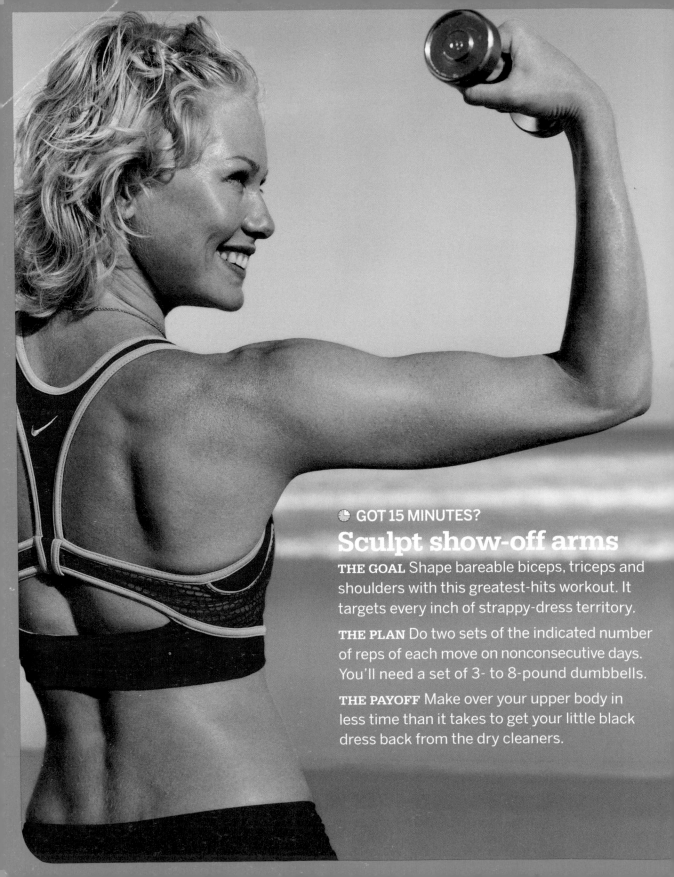

⏱ GOT 15 MINUTES?

Sculpt show-off arms

THE GOAL Shape bareable biceps, triceps and shoulders with this greatest-hits workout. It targets every inch of strappy-dress territory.

THE PLAN Do two sets of the indicated number of reps of each move on nonconsecutive days. You'll need a set of 3- to 8-pound dumbbells.

THE PAYOFF Make over your upper body in less time than it takes to get your little black dress back from the dry cleaners.

1 SNOW ANGEL

Lie facedown with arms extended out to sides, a weight in each hand a few inches off floor, palms down. Keeping legs on floor, lift chest slightly as you slowly bring arms toward legs (as shown). Lower chest as arms return to start. Do 12 reps.

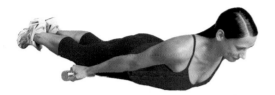

2 LATERAL RAISE

Holding weights, stand with arms down, chest lifted. Keeping right knee soft, exhale while you lift left knee as high as you can. With elbows slightly bent, inhale, then exhale as you raise arms out to sides to shoulder height (as shown). Inhale while you lower arms to start, keeping left knee lifted. Do 6 reps. Switch legs and then repeat.

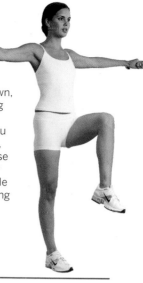

3 CLEAVAGE PUSH-UP

Kneel on all fours with knees under hips, hands aligned under head, thumbs and index fingers touching to form a diamond. Lower chest toward floor as far as you can (as shown). Push up to return to start so arms are straight but not locked; repeat. Do 12 reps.

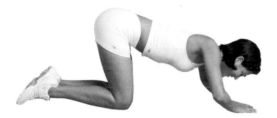

4 LAWN MOWER

Holding a weight in right hand, step left into a side lunge, left foot pointing out, right foot perpendicular to left. Rest left forearm on left thigh. Extend right arm toward front heel; pull weight diagonally up to ribs, palm facing in (as shown). Do 12 reps. Switch sides; repeat.

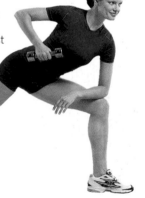

5 THE WHOLE ENCHILADA

Stand with feet hip-width apart, a weight in each hand, palms facing behind you. Keeping upper arms at sides, bend elbows and raise weights to shoulders so palms face forward, then press weights overhead. Keeping upper arms still, turn palms in and lower weights behind head until elbows are bent 90 degrees (as shown). Straighten arms and reverse sequence to complete rep. Do 12 reps.

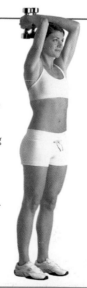

6 STORK CURL

Stand with feet hip-width apart, a weight in each hand. Shift weight to left leg and bend forward, raising right leg behind you until it's parallel to floor. Extend arms down, palms forward. Keeping upper arms still, curl dumbbells to shoulders (as shown). Lower weights. Do 6 reps. Switch legs; repeat.

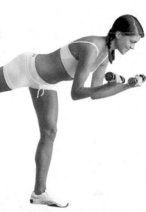

⏱ GOT 15 MINUTES?
Shoe shop smartly

THE RIGHT SNEAKER can help you exercise happily ever after. Follow these steps to find your dream match.

Before hitting the store, try this: Wet the soles of your feet and step on a dry paper towel. If you leave a C-shape print, you're a neutral runner; if you leave a ball and heel print only, you have high arches; and if the print is relatively solid with little or no indent, you have flat feet. The print dictates the type of running sneaker to buy.

NEUTRAL	HIGH ARCHES	FLAT FEET
Opt for a neutral shoe (the arches are generally less foam-filled) with a little cushioning.	Get a shoe that boasts extra cushioning; shun the one that touts extra stability.	Go for a motion-control shoe. Spot it by the denser, typically gray foam under the inside arch.

Not a runner? Zero in on a shoe made for your favorite workout. If you take the fitness class du jour, then choose a cross-trainer with a wide toe box rather than a running shoe. "A wider toe box equates to better overall balance and stability, which is important for workouts like kickboxing and cardio classes, where you do a lot of lateral movement," says Terry Schalow, product manager for the performance-running division for Asics in Irvine, California. Walkers, pick a walking-specific shoe: They have more flex in the forefoot than running sneakers to accommodate the extra time your foot spends in push-off-the-ground mode.

Whatever the shoe type, make sure you can press the top of your thumb between your big toe and the end of any sneaker you're trying on. "Your feet swell because of all the pounding from exercise," Schalow points out.

⏱ GOT 12 MINUTES?
Dress to sweat

When you take your workout outdoors, follow this checklist to avoid a fitness faux pas.

☐ **DRESS IN LAYERS,** starting with just enough to feel slightly cool—not toasty—when you step out.

☐ **SELECT A SYNTHETIC,** moisture-wicking shirt (polyester will do the trick) as your first layer. When cotton tees get sweaty, the wetness stays next to your skin and makes you prone to postworkout shivers. Your midlayer (if the temperature requires one) should also wick.

☐ **REACH FOR AN OUTER LAYER** that fits the forecast. When it's windy or drizzly but temperate, opt for a Windbreaker. If it's chilly but dry, choose a fleece. For cold, windy, wet weather, you'll need a lined, water-resistant soft-shell jacket. Add extra midlayers when it's frigid and snowy; save the down jacket for the ski slopes.

☐ **PICK SOCKS** made mainly with nylon or other synthetics. Socks with more than 50 percent cotton create more blister-making friction.

⏱ GOT 2 MINUTES?
Refresh your swimsuit

When you see broken fibers or discoloring along the center of the chest or seams of last summer's swimsuit, it's time to toss it, says Kate Rosinsky, designer for Speedo. (Also look for bagging around the body.) For a perfect-fitting one-piece, "You should be able to pull the straps as high as, but not higher than, your earlobes," Rosinsky says. "This ensures you'll have the appropriate fit around the rest of your body."

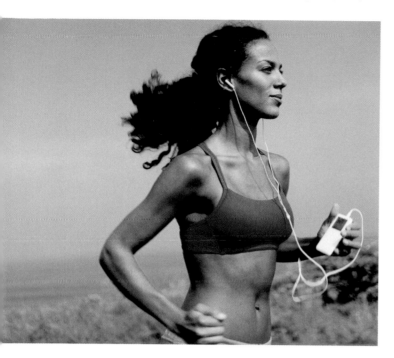

GOT 6 MINUTES?

Ban the bounce A good sports bra can reduce breast movement during exercise by up to 74 percent, a report from the University of Portsmouth in England reveals. Find your best fit with this four-point inspection.

1 **Give it the stretch test.** Grab the center of the cup with one hand and the top of the shoulder strap with the other, then pull. The less stretch, the more support. Note: You want the stretch of your straps to be in the back of the bra, not the front, where, because of the weight of your breasts, most of gravity's effects are felt.

2 **Size up straps.** Wider straps and rib bands anchor breasts better. Pick adjustable straps or bands for custom support.

3 **Consider the cups.** For smaller-breasted women, who don't need much motion control, a compression bra works well. Women with C-cups or larger may prefer the separation of individual cups.

4 **Do a jump check.** Move around the dressing room, mimicking the motion of exercise. Make sure you feel supported and that the straps don't fall. Bend forward to be certain you don't pop out.

GOT 2 MINUTES?
Lace up lightly

If you have numb feet regularly after a workout, your shoelaces may be tied too tight, explains Howard Palamarchuk, D.P.M., director of sports medicine at Temple University School of Podiatric Medicine in Philadelphia. Also try this technique: Over your arch, thread the lace from an eyelet to the one right above it, rather than making a crisscross.

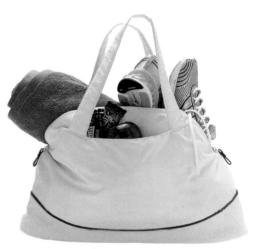

GOT 5 MINUTES?
Keep your duffel smelling sweet

The average gym bag is dark, moist, warm—an ideal home for stinky bacteria, says Kelly A. Reynolds, professor and microbiologist at the University of Arizona College of Public Health in Tucson. To avoid the sweaty-sock smell, purchase a vinyl or plastic tote (which you can wipe down weekly with a bleach-based disinfectant spray) or one with mesh pockets. Then keep your bag dry: Store dirties in a sealed plastic bag, then remove sneaks at night.

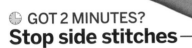

◷ GOT 2 MINUTES?
Stop side stitches

No one is quite sure what causes these pains, but some experts think they might be diaphragm cramps. To fix the glitch, slow down, breathe through pursed lips or stretch your abs—all help relax the diaphragm.

◷ GOT 1 MINUTE?
Baby your back

Preserve the natural curve of your spine during ab moves. "Instructors used to believe flattening the spine prevented strain," says SELF contributing editor Marianne Battistone, a movement therapist in New York City. "But that is stressful for your back." Start where you can barely slide fingertips under your lower back.

◷ GOT 1 MINUTE?
Breathe easy

Have walnuts as a snack. If you're among the 16 percent of people with exercise-induced asthma, then omega-3 fatty acids, in walnuts, salmon and flaxseed, may help ease your lungs, a study from Indiana University at Bloomington finds. Folks with this condition saw a 64 percent improvement in breathing by taking in 5.2 grams of omega-3s for three weeks.

◷ GOT 1 MINUTE?
Nix knee pain

If your knee joints hurt as you run but you still want to work up a sweat, switch from the pavement to a cushioned track, a treadmill or, even better, an elliptical trainer or a bike. Knees still nagging you? An upper-body ergometer— it's like a stationary bike for your arms—can provide a decent, knee-free cardio workout if you pump hard.

◷ GOT 2 MINUTES?
Feel feet relief

The magic bullet for beating sore soles may be stretching the plantar fascia (located at the base of the arch), scientists at Ithaca College in Rochester, New York, say. Doing this stretch in the A.M. relieved chronic tightness in 90 percent of exercisers: Rest the ankle of the achy foot on the opposite knee; use your hand to pull toes back toward shin. Hold 10 seconds; repeat 10 times.

YOUR GREAT-BODY TO-DON'T LIST

» **Don't look down** during squats. Instead, focus where the wall and ceiling meet to maintain proper form.

» **Don't let cardio playlists** go stale. Visit Self.com/go/music and listen to SELF's iMixes to rev yourself up!

» **Don't rack your brain** trying to remember your gym-lock combo. Get a WordLock from Magellans.com ($12), which you set using letters.

» **Don't toe-tap** as you sit. Cross your legs; trace the alphabet with your big toe one foot at a time for strong ankles.

» **Don't stay tomato-red** after a workout. Put cold water on your face to help constrict dilated blood vessels.

» **Don't do hundreds** of sit-ups. Try adding a few planks—balance in a push-up position—to firm abs faster.

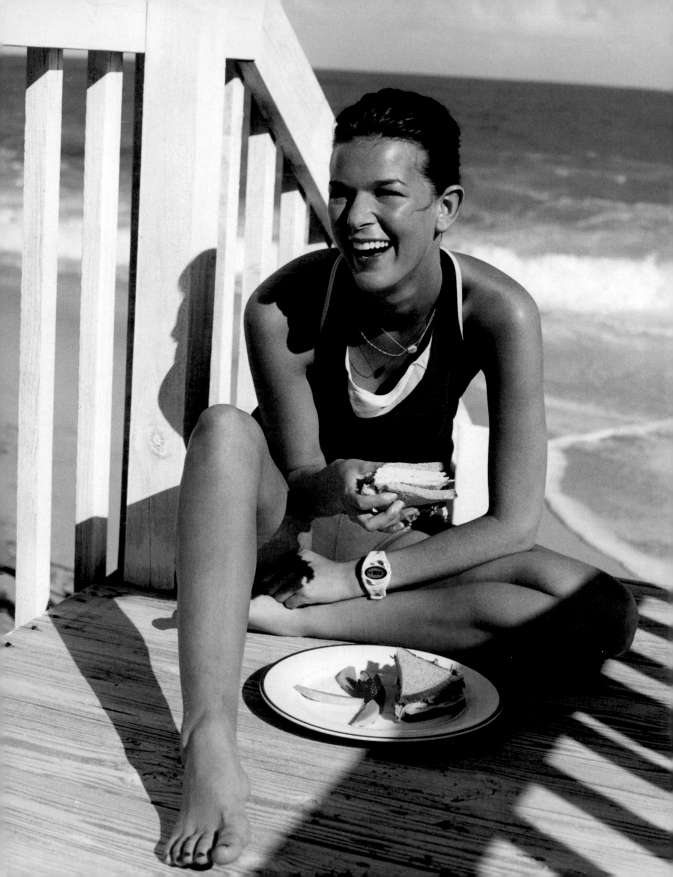

EFFORTLESS
eat-right strategies

Prepare to rejoice! From this moment on, you can forget about extreme diets, counting calories or depriving yourself of any food you love. Turn the page to begin an eat-right plan so simple and inspiring, it's guaranteed to turn even the worst junk food junkie into a healthy eater virtually overnight. Then try the easy, speedy, no-starve tips and recipes. You'll never agonize over a single bite again.

The only 10 things **you need to know to become a healthier, slimmer eater for life**

You've got the USDA telling you what to eat, the FDA preaching what not to eat, R.D.s and M.D.s chattering about RDAs and your mom looking crestfallen if you pass on the potatoes. It's enough to drive you to a plate of french fries. Help is here at last! Below, you'll find all you need to know to shop, cook and eat right for life.

1 Eat real food

Good-for-you food comes from the farm or the sea. Period. Highly processed packaged foods are linked with obesity, adult-onset diabetes and cardiovascular disease, and as these foods multiply in your diet, they displace things such as fruit and vegetables. You're better off eating a piece of cheese on wholewheat crackers than cheese-flavored chips; yogurt with berries, not ice cream with fake, fruit-flavored goop; a fruit smoothie versus a Slurpee. You get the idea.

2 Mix it up

Your body works best if you consume carbohydrates, protein and fat at every meal. Carbs provide energy and fiber; protein enhances your immune system, moves oxygen to muscles and helps your carb-fueled energy last longer; satiating fat helps your body absorb certain vitamins in everything else you eat. Make three lists: your favorite fruit and veggies, whole grains and proteins. Tack them on the fridge. Don't worry about getting enough fat; it comes along for the ride with other foods.

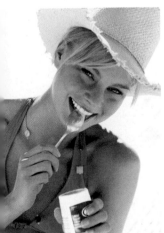

3 Slow down

A little reminder: Nobody is going to steal your meal before you're finished. Taking small forkfuls and chewing thoroughly and slowly are simple ways to lose weight. You might also take the time to arrange your food on a pretty plate and sit at the table. If you make eating an event, you'll become more mindful of the flavors and textures of the food, which encourages you to savor every bite.

4 Consume your colors

Sorry, Skittles don't count, but eating the recommended 2 cups of fruit and 2½ cups of veggies a day reduces your calorie intake (they average 100 calories per cup) and enhances immunity. The colors in fruit and vegetables come from phytonutrients; each shade safeguards a different organ. For example, the lutein in greens protects your eyes, lycopene-packed red tomatoes shield the heart and blues and purples help your brain form neurons. Keep fruit and veggies visible on your counter and the top shelf of your fridge and, like magic, you'll reach for them.

5 Splurge

Consider this a permission slip: SELF hereby decrees that [insert your name here] may eat a serving of yummy stuff when desired, and after indulging in aforementioned yummy stuff, [your name] shall not feel guilty. Deprivation never works because you continue to crave what you're missing. Try to keep it in moderation, of course, but if you do overindulge, don't sweat it. Guilt often leads to more overeating. So instead of feeling like a porker, go for a walk. Go to bed. Hit the shower and tell yourself, Oh, well. I'll do better next time. (For tasty ideas on how to indulge smartly, see "Grab a Goody" on page 80.)

6 Graze

Never allow yourself to get to the point where you feel that if you do not eat a bucket of food fast, you are going to fall over or stab someone in the eye with your stiletto heel. If you are over-hungry, you'll overeat. The alternative: Snack wisely between meals, or sub five or six smaller (300- to 350-calorie) meals for three big ones. Research shows that eating more often will reduce your appetite. Good snack options include an ounce of nuts or part-skim string cheese.

7 Read the fine print

Like some good-looking people before you get to know them, many packaged foods present a pretty face that may not reflect what's inside. The only way you'll know is if you squint at the minuscule ingredients list printed on the back. Companies must list a food's contents from largest amount to smallest; in truly whole-grain products, whole-wheat or whole-grain flour is the first ingredient, for instance. If sugar (aka sucrose, dextrose, high-fructose corn syrup) is near the top, consume the food sparingly, if at all.

8 Unplug

Women who watch three to five hours of TV a day increase their risk for obesity by 70 percent, according to a study in *The Journal of the American Medical Association.* Even two hours ups the risk by 23 percent. Why? Studies show that couch potatoes eat more sweets, red meat and refined carbohydrates, and fewer fruit and veggies, than TV teetotalers, probably because when people watch television, they're not paying attention to what they're putting into their mouth. Watch less TV and spend your newfound free time shopping for smaller clothes!

9 Sleep more

Skimp on sleep and not only do your eyelids puff up but your body might, too. When you're tired, you produce more ghrelin, a hunger-triggering hormone, and less leptin, an appetite-curbing hormone. That's why sleep-deprived people have bigger appetites and crave sweet and salty snacks. In a study from Columbia University Medical Center in New York City, researchers found adults ages 32 to 49 who slept five hours a night were 60 percent more likely to be obese than those who slept seven hours. A healthy move: Turn off your computer an hour before bedtime. Research shows that Web surfing at night impedes shut-eye. And exercise early. It takes six hours to recover; if you're cooled down, you'll fall asleep easier.

10 Don't judge

You weren't "good" today if you ate like a bunny or "bad" if you inhaled four cookies. Unless you're a cannibal, what you eat is no reflection of your moral character. Try to pick from a variety of nutritious foods. And remember, if you eat badly once in a while, you're still a good person.

🕐 GOT 10 MINUTES?

Rise and dine the smart way

If there is one meal that can make or break your weight and health, it's breakfast. A 10-year study in the journal *Lancet* shows that those who eat a morning meal consume fewer calories and less saturated fat throughout the day. Morning eaters also have flatter abs and a lower risk for heart disease than breakfast skippers. Eating anything is better than nothing, but you'll be most satisfied by a high-fiber, calcium-rich mix of whole grains, protein (including dairy) and fruit.

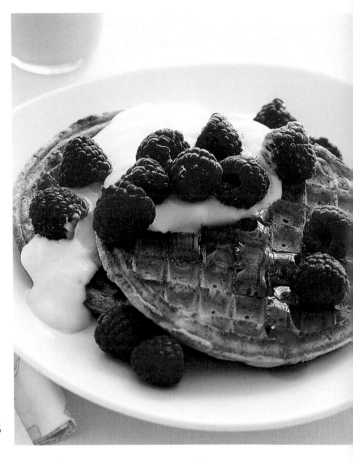

Quick 400-calorie breakfasts

MAKE IT

1 YOGURT WAFFLES
Top 2 whole-grain waffles with 1 cup lowfat plain yogurt, ½ cup raspberries, 2 tsp honey.

2 A BETTER BOWL
Mix ½ cup General Mills Fiber One bran cereal (14 g fiber) and ⅔ cup spoon-sized shredded wheat (4 g fiber); top with 2 tbsp nuts and 1 cup skim milk. Or try Kashi GoLean (10 g fiber per ¾ cup).

3 SPICY BREAKFAST BURRITO Scramble 2 egg whites and 1 yolk in skillet coated with cooking spray; add a dash of dried chipotle chile and 1 tbsp salsa. Warm a 6-inch whole-wheat tortilla in the oven or on a griddle and fill with scrambled eggs; add ¼ cup shredded romaine and roll into a burrito. Enjoy with 1 cup of cubed fresh melon (any variety) and 1 cup skim milk on the side.

4 FRUITY OATMEAL
Top 1 cup cooked oatmeal with 1 cup raspberries or ½ cup blueberries or an apple, sliced; 2 tbsp chopped nuts; 1 tsp brown sugar or honey. Serve with 1 cup skim milk.

TAKE IT

5 FAST FOOD Stop at McDonald's for scrambled eggs, English muffin (toss half), sliced apples and an 8-oz container of lowfat milk.

6 DELI NOSH Order a toasted whole-wheat English muffin or 2 slices whole-wheat toast; top with 1 tbsp peanut butter. Have with 1 pear or apple and 1 cup skim milk.

7 BREAKFAST BAR
Read the nutrition label before you take a bite. Look for one with at least 2 g fiber, and check that *whole grains* or *bran* is the first ingredient listed.

🕐 GOT 1 MINUTE?
Go halfsies to break a sugar habit

Can't give up your morning fix of sweet cereal? Make a 50-50 blend with a whole-grain variety. You'll slash calories, fat and sugar but not a lick of taste. Gradually shift portions until you're eating mostly the good stuff; when you're ready, complete the switch. Easy!

🕐 GOT 5 MINUTES?
Brew up a cup of good health

Green tea has the healthiest rep, but research shows that the black variety contains more disease-fighting antioxidants. No matter which kind you like, use boiling water and allow tea to steep 5 minutes to release the most antioxidants.

🕐 GOT 3 MINUTES?
Buy a better egg

ONCE CRUELLY BANISHED because of their high cholesterol content, eggs have scrambled back onto our plates. Maybe it's because the news has spread that eggs contain nearly 25 percent less cholesterol than was previously thought. Plus, scientists now know that cholesterol-containing foods normally don't raise heart disease risk in healthy people (unlike foods with too much saturated fat, so skip the bacon). A study in the journal *Metabolism* found that eating up to three eggs daily doesn't elevate LDL, the harmful form of cholesterol. Best of all, eggs are protein powerhouses, helping you stay full. Check out the egg options, below, which offer a variety of perks—and get cracking!

EGG TYPE	NUTRITION FACTS	BODY BENEFIT
Regular	74 calories per egg 5 g fat 1.6 g saturated fat	All eggs pack 6 g of satiating protein, which helps you feel satisfied. White and brown eggs are nutritional equals.
Omega-3 enriched	70 calories per egg 4.5 g fat 1.5 g saturated fat	Omega-3 fatty acids help keep your heart healthy and reduce the risk for heart attack.
Organic	74 calories per egg 5 g fat 1.6 g saturated fat	Hens are not given hormones or antibiotics, which, in turn, reduces your own exposure to them.
Liquid	45 calories per ¼ cup serving 2 g fat 0.5 g saturated fat	These egg subs are made with only whites, so they're great if you're trying to lose weight. Some provide omega-3s and added nutrients.

🕐 GOT 15 MINUTES?
Savor the ideal noon meal

YOUR LIFE INBOX may be so stuffed with to do's that eating an actual lunch feels as if it's an unattainable luxury. But what you save in time you end up losing in productivity. If you don't feed your body every four hours or so, your blood sugar level will dip, resulting in a diminished ability to focus and concentrate. Not exactly the prescription for an energized afternoon! So grab a nutritious bite—sit down and enjoy it if you can, get it on the go if you must. To keep you satisfied, your lunch should have 450 to 600 calories and contain a mix of whole grains (such as brown rice, quinoa or whole-wheat bread), about 3 oz lean protein (such as fish, chicken or turkey breast, egg whites or beans) and some healthy fat (such as 1 tbsp olive oil on your salad). Any less and you'll be raiding the candy stash by 3 P.M.; if you eat more, you'll feel stuffed and sluggish. Here are three quickie ways to put whole grains, protein and fat together:

● Heat 1½ cups canned lentil soup with 2 hefty handfuls of spinach leaves tossed in for extra nutrition and flavor; enjoy with 1 slice whole-grain bread and 1 oz hard cheese (such as colby, Swiss or cheddar).

● Spread 2 slices whole-grain bread with 1 tbsp lowfat mayo; layer on ¼ cup arugula, 2 slices tomato, 2 oz chicken or turkey breast and 1 slice Swiss cheese. Pair with 1 cup V8 or skim milk and an apple.

● Fill a warmed, whole-wheat tortilla with ¾ cup canned, rinsed black or pinto beans, ¼ cup reduced-fat shredded cheddar or Mexican cheese blend, 1 cup sliced red or green bell pepper and ¼ cup prepared or fresh tomato salsa. Hot sauce is optional. ¡Olé!

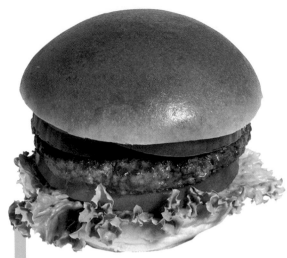

🕐 GOT 10 MINUTES?
Have lunch on the go

Each fast-food lunch here offers a decent dose of satiating protein, plus most come in around 400 calories or less. Add a piece of fresh fruit or 1 cup skim milk to bump up calories and satisfaction.

● Wendy's Mandarin Chicken Salad with ⅓ packet Oriental Sesame Dressing

● McDonald's Cheeseburger (regular size) with Caesar salad (no chicken) and ½ packet Newman's Own Low Fat Balsamic Vinaigrette (and hold the fries!)

● Panera Bread Grilled Salmon Salad

● Au Bon Pain Jamaican Black Bean Soup and a piece of French Country White Bread (skip the butter)

● Subway 6 Inch Turkey Breast Sandwich

🕐 GOT 3 MINUTES?
Banish lunch boredom

Break out of your lunch rut by asking a coworker to swap healthy brown-bag meals. One easy option: a whole-wheat pita stuffed with ⅓ cup hummus, 1 oz mozzarella, a little fresh parsley and lettuce; pair with 3 cups greens tossed with olive oil and lemon juice.

⏱ GOT 5 MINUTES?
Build a better salad

You'd think that eating salad was a no-brainer diet move, but most salad bars feature so many fat bombs that you'd be better off with sausage pizza (well, nearly). To put together the light yet satisfying salad you want, start with the darkest possible greens—they're rich in nutrients. (Iceberg lettuce is water masquerading as a vegetable.) The best picks are spinach, watercress and arugula; pile on other leaves you like for color and bulk. Then add 3 to 4 oz lean protein, such as beans, grilled chicken, tofu or shrimp. The protein is key to creating a mealworthy salad because it's filling. And keep your taste buds interested with creative and nutritious add-ins:

Fix

- ☐ **ALMONDS** Rich in fiber and healthy fats
- ☐ **ARTICHOKE HEARTS** Contain vitamin C, folate, potassium, magnesium and fiber
- ☐ **BAKED PLANTAIN CHIPS** Low-calorie and high in potassium and vitamin C
- ☐ **BELL PEPPERS** Red ones are loaded with vitamin C.
- ☐ **CAULIFLOWER** Lots of fiber; good source of folate
- ☐ **DRIED CRANBERRIES OR CHERRIES** Chewy sweetness, plus potassium and vitamin A
- ☐ **FIGS** One of the highest-fiber fruits
- ☐ **PEAS** Contain vitamins A and C, iron and potassium; try wasabi-roasted peas for a spicy punch.
- ☐ **PISTACHIOS** One of the highest-fiber nuts
- ☐ **PUMPKIN SEEDS** Contain protein, B vitamins, iron
- ☐ **QUINOA** Boasts the highest protein content of all grains
- ☐ **STEAMED, SHELLED EDAMAME** For a boost of protein, calcium, iron, zinc and B vitamins

Nix

- ☐ **A LADLEFUL OF DRESSING** A quarter cup of blue cheese dressing could add 6 g of artery-clogging saturated fat. Try 1 tbsp of heart-friendly olive oil and as much vinegar as you want instead.
- ☐ **CRISPY ANYTHING** Noodles, chicken, fish, whatever. Crispy equals fried equals fatty.
- ☐ **COLD PASTA DISHES** They seem innocent enough but are usually mixed with gobs of mayo, oil or both.
- ☐ **DISHES MIXED WITH MAYONNAISE** Mayo adds 11 g fat and 100 calories per tbsp to whatever it touches.
- ☐ **HOT ENTRÉES** If you didn't make it, you don't know the ingredients or the calorie count.
- ☐ **MARINATED VEGGIES** A little oil is healthy, but these are usually swamped in the stuff, adding lots of calories.

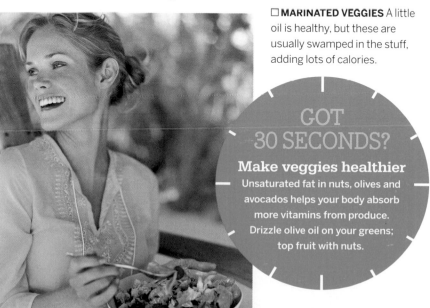

GOT 30 SECONDS?
Make veggies healthier
Unsaturated fat in nuts, olives and avocados helps your body absorb more vitamins from produce. Drizzle olive oil on your greens; top fruit with nuts.

⏱ GOT 15 MINUTES?

Serve a healthy evening meal

When it comes to eating dinner, many of us fall into one of two extremes: We either eat far too much or we bypass it altogether. Both approaches can backfire, causing weight gain. Skipping dinner slows your metabolism, so you burn fewer calories throughout the day; by not eating, you also deprive your system of the essential fuel it needs to repair and rebuild cells, muscles and digestive enzymes while you sleep. And if you have too many calories at night, you risk weight gain because you're unlikely to burn them off before bed. A big dinner can interfere with sleep, as well. Instead, have a balanced meal of around 500 calories, and finish up eating at least two hours before your bedtime.

Cook it With these simple recipes, you'll serve up a tasty 550-calorie dinner in a flash.

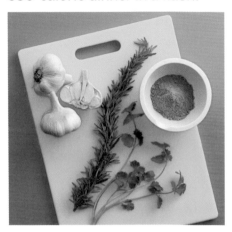

Call for it Takeout is easy, but dialing for dinner can deliver more than a meal—entrées can easily hit 1,200 calories! Stay slim with these tasty options.

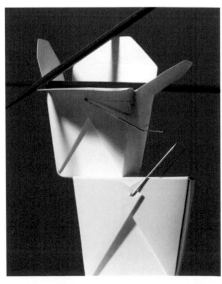

Wok star

Stir-fry 1½ cups broccoli in 2 tsp canola oil with 1 tsp each chopped garlic and ginger. Add 4 oz firm tofu (or shrimp); stir until hot. Add 3 tbsp water; 2 tsp soy sauce, a pinch of sugar. Simmer until done; remove from heat. Top with 1 tbsp chopped cashews. Serve with 1 cup brown rice.

Fast fish

Mix 4 tsp olive oil with 2½ tsp lemon juice. Brush 4 oz salmon with 1 tbsp lemon oil; dust with dill. Broil 8 minutes. Toss 3 cups sliced veggies in rest of lemon oil. Serve with 2 slices whole-grain bread sprinkled with 2 tsp each olive oil and Parmesan, and garlic to taste.

Quickie chicken

Slice ¼ rotisserie chicken (white or dark meat, skin removed). Serve with a large microwaved sweet potato sliced in ½-inch rounds and dressed with 1 tsp trans fat–free margarine and 2 tbsp lowfat plain yogurt. Serve with a salad made with 3 cups mixed greens and 1 cup cherry tomatoes tossed with 1 tbsp plus 1½ tsp regular salad dressing.

Perfect pasta

Cook ¾ cup dry whole-wheat penne; heat ½ cup marinara and ½ cup precooked skinless chicken breast; combine. Sprinkle with 1 tbsp Parmesan. Serve with 3 cups mixed greens and 75 calories' worth of salad dressing.

Chinese

3 SMART PICKS
- Hot-and-sour soup
  110 calories,
  4 g fat per cup
- Hunan tofu and brown rice
  206 calories,
  7 g fat per cup
- Mandarin chicken
  364 calories,
  15 g fat per cup

3 EAT-SLIM TRICKS
- Steer clear of sweet-and-sour entrées; they tend to be deep-fried and fatty.
- Dish out food with a fork to drain excess sauce, a prime source of fat and calories.
- Use chopsticks; you'll eat more slowly.

Italian

3 SMART PICKS
- Tomato, mozzarella and basil salad
  196 calories, 14 g fat per average-sized side order
- Thin-crust cheese and vegetable pizza
  170 calories,
  6 g fat per slice
- Linguine with marinara sauce
  450 calories, 9 g fat per average entrée

3 EAT-SLIM TRICKS
- Get parmigiana dishes baked (no breading)
- Trade in a meat entrée and a side of pasta for pasta with meat sauce.
- Go for tomato sauces instead of cream ones.

Mexican

3 SMART PICKS
- Beef taquitos
  63 calories,
  3 g fat each
- Chicken flautas
  65 calories,
  4 g fat each
- Fish tacos
  235 calories,
  4 g fat each

3 EAT-SLIM TRICKS
- Flavor your food with tomatillo sauce, not fatty sour cream or guacamole.
- Ask for raw vegetables instead of sautéed when ordering fajitas.
- Request black beans in place of the refried beans typically served with entrées.

Diner

3 SMART PICKS
- Vegetarian chili
  205 calories,
  1 g fat per cup
- Barbecue chicken breast
  300 calories, 10 g fat per 6-oz serving
- Roast beef on whole-wheat bread
  459 calories,
  12 g fat

3 EAT-SLIM TRICKS
- Skip mayo-heavy sides like coleslaw. Opt for fruit salad.
- Ask for double the veggies and half the meat in wraps.
- Craving greasy spoon? Order chicken fingers from the kids' menu.

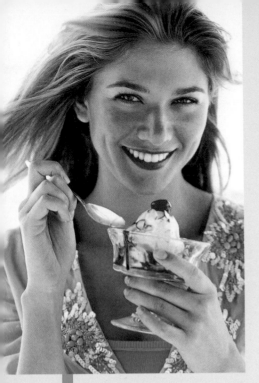

🕐 GOT 1 MINUTE? Grab a goody

Not only is snacking fun but it's actually helpful as part of a healthy, balanced diet. Savvy snacking can even help you lose weight by staving off hunger pangs and overeating. But most of us snack too much, with an astonishing 26 percent of our calories sneaking in between meals. According to the USDA, if you are not trying to lose weight, you can spend about 265 calories a day on snacks. (Scale that back to no more than 160 if dieting.) Ideally, you will nosh on fresh fruit, nutritious vegetables and calcium-rich lowfat yogurt, but if the rest of your diet is sound, there is plenty of room for a treat, too. Every munchie here comes in at or under 200 calories. Pick your favorite and enjoy!

Craving salty?	Calories
5 olives (any kind)	45
1 small Martin's pretzel	50
2 oz Applegate Honey and Maple Turkey Breast wrapped around 2 bread-and-butter pickles	80
¼ cup hummus, 3 carrot sticks	80
1 Laughing Cow Light Swiss Original wedge, 3 Kavli Crispy Thin crackers	85
3 cups air-popped popcorn	90
1 oz buffalo mozzarella, ½ cup cherry or grape tomatoes	94
1 bag Baked! Cheetos 100 Calorie Mini Bites	100
15 Eden's Nori Maki Crackers rice crackers	110
1 cup unshelled edamame	120
50 Eden's Vegetable Chips	130
¼ cup Trader Joe's Chili con Queso, 18 baked tortilla chips	140
½ cup pumpkin seeds in shell	143
15 cashew or pecan halves	150
2 pieces (30 g) prosciutto, 4 dried figs	154
20 shoestring french fries	200

Craving sweet?	Calories
1 package Original Apple Nature Valley Fruit Crisps	50
9 animal crackers	90
10 gummi bears	100
10 dried pineapple pieces	100
1 Starbucks Mocha Frappuccino bar	120
1 package Back to Nature Honey Graham Sticks	120
½ banana rolled in 1 tbsp frozen semisweet chocolate chips	123
2 tbsp Better 'n Peanut Butter, 4 stalks celery	124
1 bag Orville Redenbacher's Smart Pop Butter Mini Bags topped with a spritz of butter spray and 1 tsp sugar	126
24 Annie's Chocolate Chip Bunny Graham cookies	140
Half of a 1.08-oz container of M&M's Minis mixed with ⅓ cup lowfat granola	145
1 McDonald's Fruit 'n Yogurt Parfait	160
3 original Oreos	160
1 container Fage Greek Total 2% fat yogurt, 2 tsp honey	173

⏱ GOT 5 MINUTES?

Lose extra liquid calories

A nondiet soda packs around 160 calories; a fancy coffee drink or fruit smoothie can easily exceed 500. Keep everyday sips from slipping you up with these strategies:

CHECK LABELS Can't find one on your cup? Visit the company website. Starbucks, Jamba Juice and other chains list their nutrition facts online.

SIP PLAIN OLD WATER Unless you're a triathlete, you don't need energy drinks to stay hydrated. Nor are fortified drinks the solution. They may sound healthy, but some can have as many as 125 calories per bottle. Water works just fine.

LIGHTEN UP Easy calorie controller: Go for flavored drinks with no more than 10 calories per 8-oz serving, such as low- or no-calorie teas.

RESET YOUR ALARM CLOCK If you're rested, you won't need that midday supersized, super fattening coffee drink to stay awake the rest of the afternoon.

⏱ GOT 2 MINUTES?
Stash nutritious nibbles

The next time you're grocery shopping, pick up a few satisfying bites (200 calories or less) to keep within easy reach.

● Satisfy an urge to crunch with 1-oz packs of sunflower seeds (or portion into sealable bags) and stick them in a desk drawer: They're protein-rich to help offset drowsiness (180 calories).

● Load your gym bag with healthy carbs, such as 3 graham cracker sheets (165 calories) or ⅓ cup dried fruit (134 calories).

● In your car, stock nongreasy granola bars (120 calories) or almonds (12 are about 80 calories). Park before eating!

⏱ GOT 3 MINUTES?
Freshen up your H_2O

Craving flavor? Skip high-calorie drinks and fix a tray of fruity cubes: Pour 1½ cups pure cran-raspberry juice into an ice-cube tray, drop 2 or 3 frozen berries into each cube and freeze. Each cube provides 10 percent of your daily vitamin C needs and turns water into a delicious drink, all for only 13 calories.

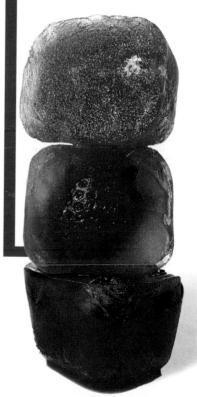

⏱ GOT 12 MINUTES (OR LESS)? Fix a fast, healthy bite

PUMP IRON WITH A PITA PIZZA

Make (and eat!) a cheesy, nutritious personal pie for only 309 calories.

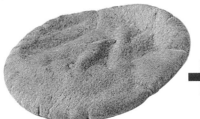

DRIZZLE 1 tsp olive oil over a whole-grain pita.

+

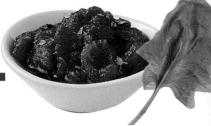

ADD ¼ cup canned diced tomato with basil. Sprinkle on ¼ cup torn fresh spinach leaves.

SHAKE UP YOUR SALSA

This appetizer offers vitamin C and heart-friendly fat for 300 calories per serving.

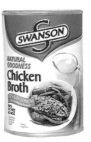

SLICE, score and peel 1 mango.

+

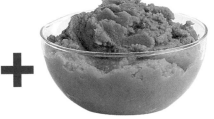

PIT, peel and dice 1 Hass avocado.

SOUP UP YOUR SOUP

For a slim 159 calories, you'll get more than 100 percent of your daily A and C.

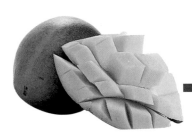

HEAT a 14-oz can fat-free chicken broth over medium-high heat.

+

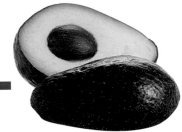

BLEND IN a 15-oz can pumpkin puree using a whisk.

SAVOR A LIGHT FONDUE

The delicious treat is only 252 calories per serving (it feeds 8). Go ahead, invite friends over!

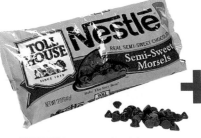

HEAT 1⅓ cups semisweet chocolate chips over low heat.

+

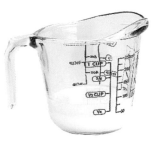

ADD ⅓ cup nonfat evaporated milk; stir; add ⅓ cup skim milk.

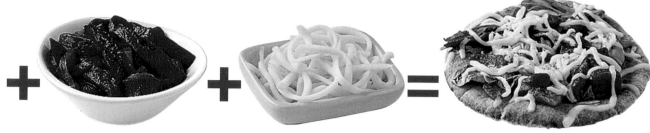

LAYER ¼ cup prepared roasted red peppers over spinach.

TOP with ¼ cup shredded part-skim mozzarella.

BROIL for 4 minutes or until cheese has melted. *Mangia!*

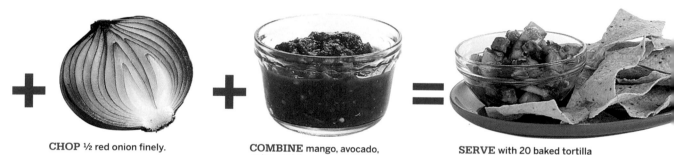

CHOP ½ red onion finely.

COMBINE mango, avocado, onion and 4 oz prepared salsa.

SERVE with 20 baked tortilla chips for you and a friend.

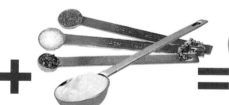
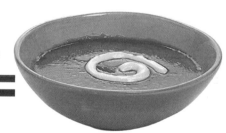

POUR 1 cup orange juice into saucepan and stir 3 minutes.

ADD 1 tbsp light sour cream, ¼ tsp nutmeg, ¼ tsp salt, ⅛ tsp pepper.

SPOON into 2 bowls; garnish with 1 tsp light sour cream.

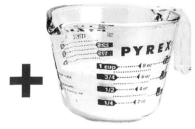
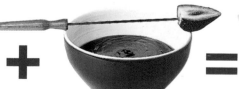
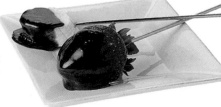

BLEND IN ¾ cup powdered sugar; stir until smooth.

TRANSFER to a fondue pot. Use a bowl if you don't have a set.

SERVE with 3 cups each strawberries and banana slices.

🕐 GOT 1 MINUTE?
Give yourself permission to indulge. (We mean it!)

Even if you're trying to lose weight, it's smart to make room for dessert now and then. Skipping it altogether may make you feel deprived, and denying yourself something you really want can increase cravings. You can spend some or all of your daily snack calories on a goody, or save up calories over a few days' time to spend on a big treat like a sundae. Reminder: Most young women can afford to eat about 265 calories' worth of snacks and/or desserts a day (about 160 if you're dieting). The best news? Choose with care and you can satisfy your sweet tooth without blowing your diet.

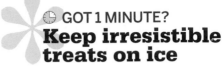

🕐 GOT 1 MINUTE?
Keep irresistible treats on ice

Your freezer may become your best diet buddy: Freeze single servings of must-have bites (Fun Size candy bars, for instance); they take a long time to finish, so you'll be satisfied long before you even think of reaching for seconds.

🕐 GOT 3 MINUTES?
Eat what you want

Craving something fatty? Give in. A study from Brown University Medical School in Providence, Rhode Island, reports that people who ate the same cake four days in a row found it less appealing and were able to resist. Have a little of a favorite treat regularly and you may stop craving it.

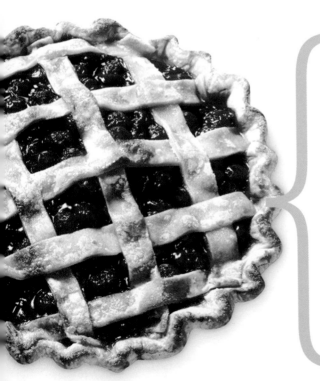

🕐 GOT 7 MINUTES?
Hit your 9-a-day goal with dessert

Enjoy a 5-oz portion of apple crisp or cherry pie (made with fruit juice) and you can check off one of your daily servings of fruit. Five oz of blueberry tart counts as roughly two thirds of a fruit serving. Or savor 5 oz of banana bread or peach cobbler and you've satisfied the requirement for about half a serving of fruit. For a light bite, try a piece of naturally lowfat angel food cake with ½ cup of strawberries (one fruit serving). So go ahead, order dessert—and hold the guilt.

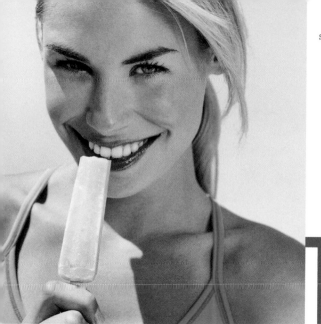

🕐 GOT 5 MINUTES?
Get in every last lick

Nothing says summer like ice pops or a scoop of ice cream (even if it's snowing!). Light versions so tasty you'd never guess they weren't the real thing:

BEST POPS

Less than 200 calories	Calories	Fat
Tofutti Hooray! Hooray! Soy Bars, chocolate and vanilla	150	9 g
Tropicana Real Fruit, orange and cream	80	2.5 g
Klondike Slim-a-Bear, fudge	90	1.5 g
Edy's Whole Fruit, strawberry	80	0 g
No Sugar Added Fudgsicles	40	1 g

BEST LOWFAT ICE CREAMS

Less than 175 calories	Calories	Fat
Starbucks Low Fat Latte Ice Cream	170	3 g
Dreyer's/Edy's Slow Churned Light Peanut Butter Cup	130	6 g
Dreyer's/Edy's Slow Churned Light Mint Chocolate Chip	120	4.5 g
Friendly's Smooth Churned Light Vanilla Ice Cream	100	3.5 g

MAKE A FRESH FRUIT POP This one has only 124 calories and is loaded with fiber. For two: Peel a banana; cut in half. Slide a stick into each piece. Dip in 2 oz nonfat yogurt; roll in mix of 1 tbsp wheat germ, 1 tbsp chopped almonds. Freeze in wax paper.

🕐 GOT 6 MINUTES?
Enjoy a chocolate high

INDULGING IN ANYTHING pleasurable can spike immunity. Merely inhaling the scent of chocolate does the job; your brain thinks a mouthful is imminent. Why disappoint it? Choose wisely and your chocolate treat will also improve your heart health. Some types of chocolate are rich in antioxidant superstars called flavonols, yet others are a bust; the way the cacao (yep, that's the correct spelling) bean is processed will make or break a product's flavonol content. Be sure your next chocolate fix is healthy:

● Pass on products that contain alkali or Dutch-processed cocoa; these terms indicate the beans were prepared using a process known as Dutching, which reduces the flavonols.
● Opt for dark chocolate; milk is more diluted with milk and sugar, reducing flavonols.
● Make your own hot cocoa. A cup made from natural, unsweetened cocoa may be higher in flavonols and fiber than chocolate bars.

HEARTY HOT CHOCOLATE
Serves 2
¼ cup plus 3 tbsp unsweetened cocoa powder
1 tbsp plus 1 tsp sugar
2 cups skim milk

Whisk cocoa powder and sugar in a small saucepan. Whisk in milk; heat over medium-low heat, stirring until sugar dissolves, about 1 minute. Increase heat to medium; stir until steam rises, about 4 minutes. Do not boil. Pour into 2 mugs.
155 calories, 2.6 g fat per serving

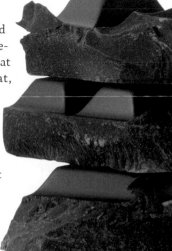

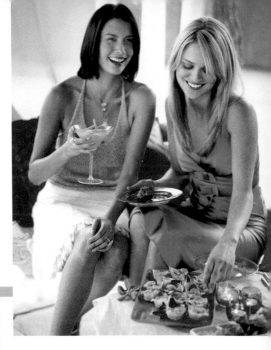

⏱ GOT 1 MINUTE?
Knock hundreds of calories off dinner

IT'S EASIER THAN ever to overeat these days: In the past 20 years, dine-out dishes have ballooned by as much as 500 percent as restaurants offer more food to lure budget-conscious consumers, a study in the *American Journal of Public Health* reports. Add a drink and a roll from the bread basket, and one meal out can equal a whole day's worth of calories! Fortunately, you can eat out and have fun without overdoing it.

ASK YOUR SERVER TO REMOVE THE BREAD BASKET and bring a raw veggie sampler instead; some eateries will do this, gratis. Or crunch on a bread stick.

FOLLOW THE RULE OF TWO Scan the menu's drinks, appetizers, entrées and desserts, then order any two you want (i.e., one drink and one entrée). You'll feel indulged but will keep your calories under control.

CHOOSE SOMETHING DIFFERENT If you always get "the usual" at your favorite haunt, you may be in for more than a mouthful. We eat bigger portions of foods we eat often, show studies at Cornell University in Ithaca, New York. Get off autopilot and try a new dish.

REQUEST A SECOND CANDLE Dim light makes you feel uninhibited, and research shows people who dine under soft lighting underestimate their calorie intake more so than those noshing under brighter lights. If you can, choose a well-lit table rather than a secluded booth. When you're out in the open you'll be more aware of how much you're eating.

GOT 30 SECONDS?
Eat less automatically
Wave off the waiter when he tries to clear plates. People who saw evidence of how much they'd eaten ate 27 percent less than those with a midmeal busing.

⏱ GOT 3 MINUTES?
Plan a healthy (and fun) night out

You're on the town with the girls. If you're not careful, wine, appetizers, a huge entrée and dessert will all vanish before you realize how stuffed you are. Be aware of the tendency to eat more when you're with a group: For one thing, the variety of appetizers stimulates a surge of dopamine, a brain chemical associated with reward and motivation. Your brain says, "Yum. Feed me more!" Second, conversation distracts you from the amount of food you're eating. Keep in control by ordering a light soup or green salad while the others attack the appetizers, and get a glass of water so you have something to sip along with your wine; spring for sparkling to make it feel special. If you can, read the menu online beforehand so you can pick out the healthiest dishes to order. Eat mindfully, and gauge your hunger periodically throughout the meal, stopping when you've had enough. And arrive with a plan for dessert. If you're going to want it, adjust your order to leave room.

⏱ GOT 2 MINUTES? Pick a great wine

A glass of wine turns dinner out into a celebration—and at about 135 calories per 6-oz glass, wine is a diet bargain compared with mixed drinks, which can hit 400 calories. (It's healthy, too: Red and even white wines contain substances that can reduce the risk for heart disease.) Use our cheat sheet below to pair the perfect vino with any light meal. *Salut!*

MEAL	YOU'RE HAVING	POUR
Brunch	Whole-grain waffles with maple syrup or powdered sugar and raspberries	Italian Brachetto d'Acqui, a sparkling red with a hint of sugar. The subtle sweetness of the wine complements the tartness of the berries.
Lunch	Chilled soup, such as gazpacho	A Spanish dry white such as Albariño or Txakoli, a slightly fizzy, lower-alcohol white from the northern part of Spain. Both are well balanced and taste similar to Riesling.
	Salad with a vinaigrette dressing	A high-acid wine such as a fruity New Zealand Sauvignon Blanc that can stand up to any dressing. Add nuts, smoked turkey, cheese or fruit to your salad; wine will go better with these ingredients.
Dinner	Stir-fry of veggies and tofu	A light-bodied Pinot Grigio, a crisp rosé or a Pinot Noir go well with soy sauce–infused entrées. Tannic reds such as Syrah are too overwhelming.
	Sushi	If you're tired of sake, try Champagne, which won't compete with the delicate flavor of raw fish. When in doubt, order Champagne. It goes with everything!

⏱ GOT 1 MINUTE?
Reenergize to beat a hangover

Oops! Last night may have been a little *too* fun—you're headachy, starving and thirsty, signs of dehydration and low blood sugar. Give your body what it needs by drinking water and boosting blood sugar with fresh fruit such as cantaloupe or oranges. And take a nap!

GOT 2 MINUTES?
Suss out supermarket sushi

Surprise: The rolls in the supermarket may be safer than those at your favorite Asian eatery, because grocery stores generally adhere to rigorous state and internal safety standards. Check that the thermostat is set lower than 41 degrees, and sushi is below the cooler's fill line; if it smells fishy or citrusy (a tip-off it's been doused in lemon juice to cover a foul odor), pass.

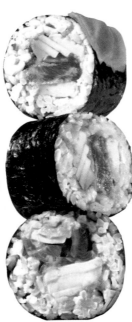

GOT 3 MINUTES?
Get smart about organic produce

ORGANIC FRUIT and veggies cost more, but are they worth it? It depends: Not all conventionally grown picks are high in pesticides. Avoid only the most contaminated varieties, and you'll cut your pesticide exposure by 90 percent.

BUY ORGANIC	REGULAR IS FINE
● Apples	● Asparagus
● Bell peppers	● Avocados
● Celery	● Bananas
● Cherries	● Broccoli
● Grapes (imported)	● Cabbage
● Lettuce	● Kiwis
● Nectarines	● Onions
● Peaches	● Pineapples
● Pears	● Sweet peas (frozen)
● Potatoes	● Sweet corn (frozen)
● Spinach	
● Strawberries	

GOT 5 MINUTES?
Choose fresh fish wisely

THE FDA ADVISES young women who are now pregnant or who are thinking about becoming pregnant to avoid exposure to fish high in mercury. But because fish is rich in healthy, heart-helping fats, the agency does recommend enjoying up to 12 oz of low-mercury fish a week. The best low-mercury choices are catfish, cod, crab, fish sticks, flounder, halibut, lobster, mahimahi, salmon, scallops, shrimp, sole, tilapia and trout. Canned tuna, red snapper and sea bass are OK to eat occasionally. Avoid blue marlin, king mackerel, orange roughy, shark, swordfish, tilefish and tuna steak. Look for these clues to the freshest catch:

A POPULAR MARKET Stores that have a high turnover in their offerings generally offer a better selection.

GOOD PRESENTATION Whole fish and fillets should be on ice and should be free of fishy smells.

OVERALL SHINE Whole fish should have bright, clear eyes and smooth, gleaming scales. Steaks and fillets should look moist and have an even coloring. Brown spots or tiny tears in the flesh can signal age.

FIRMNESS The flesh of a whole fish should bounce back when you push on it through plastic. If it doesn't, it's past its peak and should be thrown back.

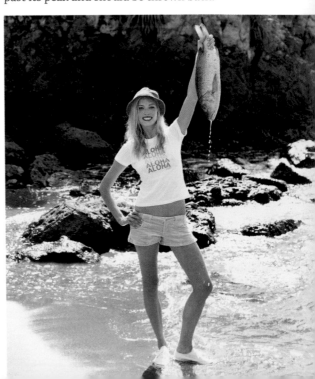

⊕ GOT 1 MINUTE?

Buy the best beef Lean red meat can fit into any healthy diet. Here's how to enjoy it your way.

LABEL	WHAT IT MEANS	BODY BENEFIT
Natural	Cows eat grain. No added preservatives; may have added hormones and antibiotics. This is basic, factory-farmed Grade A beef.	As with all beef, it's rich in zinc, iron and protein. "Natural" refers to how it's processed (minimally), not raised.
Organic	Cows graze and eat organic feed. No preservatives, added hormones or antibiotics. This is the only government-regulated term.	You reduce your own exposure to antibiotic-resistant bacteria and risk for E. coli.
Grass-fed	Cows chomp only on grass. This variety of beef usually doesn't have preservatives, hormones or antibiotics.	Highest in heart-healthy omega-3 fatty acids, thanks to the diet; grass-fed beef also tends to be the leanest.
Farm-fresh	Local farmers can explain precisely how they raise their herd (organic, grass-fed or both).	You get exactly what you want. Find a farmers' market at AMS.USDA.gov.

⊕ GOT 3 MINUTES?
Clean your veggies

Water won't wash off bacteria that causes food poisoning, so disinfect with this trick: Fill a spray bottle with white vinegar and another with 3 percent hydrogen peroxide. Spray produce with vinegar, then peroxide. Rinse well with water. (You can't wash off some pesticides at all; for buying tips, see list, at left.)

⊕ GOT 1 MINUTE?
Check your chicken

● Give a raw breast a push with your finger; the flesh should be very firm and not slimy. Look for a little fat on the breast, which should be white. If it's yellow, don't buy it.
● Organic chicken (it cuts your exposure to antibiotic-resistant bacteria) is pink when raw, white cooked. Conventional birds are yellower.

⊕ GOT 1 MINUTE?
Take your food's temperature

To reduce your risk of food poisoning, always cook your meats to proper temperatures. That means:

THE MEAT	INTERNAL TEMPERATURE
Beef hamburger	160
Beef roasts/steaks: medium-rare	145
well-done	170
Poultry: ground chicken, turkey	165
boneless turkey roast	170
poultry breast	170
whole chicken, turkey	180
thighs, wings, drumstick	180
Stuffing	165
Pork, all cuts: medium	160
well-done	170
Ham: fresh, raw	160
cooked, reheated	140

Note When meat, poultry or fish is charred, it forms a compound that may cause cancer. Cook to medium, rather than well-done; marinate to further reduce risk. If charring does occur, trim it off and eat the rest.

⏱ GOT 15 MINUTES (OR LESS)?

Lose weight painlessly No calorie counting, no deprivation, no kidding! Each day for the next 14 days, try one simple weight loss tip; if you like that tip, stick with it. Not for you? Move on. In two weeks, you'll make over your eating habits in a naturally slimming way that fits your lifestyle—a surefire formula for long-term success.

⑤ MIN Take in more fiber

Have two foods with at least 3 g fiber per serving today. Studies suggest that we absorb up to 6 percent fewer calories when we follow a high-fiber diet that includes at least 34 g a day. Fiber is filling and helps stabilize blood sugar levels, which may prevent binges. Toss ¼ cup beans on your salad (4 g), snack on an unpeeled apple (3.3 g) or order a baked sweet potato (3.4 g) to have with dinner.

⑮ MIN Quit the clean-plate club

Choose your usual foods and drinks, but have only 80 percent of every serving and leave the rest on your plate or in your glass. You'll cut about 350 calories a day, which could translate into a loss of 30 pounds in a year, all without depriving yourself of the things you love. Store the set-aside portions from home-cooked meals and save them for a snack. Eating out? Ask the waiter to pack up 20 percent of the dish in a take-out container before you begin eating.

⑩ MIN Have more protein

Many dieters skip protein-rich food, such as dairy products, in their effort to cut calories. But your body actually expends more energy digesting protein than fat or carbs—talk about an effortless calorie burn! In addition, high-protein foods can delay hunger pains and bolster your energy. Aim to eat about 50 g protein throughout the day, and focus on sources that are low in fat (they'll be lighter in calories, too). Good choices include 6 oz nonfat plain yogurt (9 g), 4 oz baked salmon fillet (25 g) or a roasted chicken breast (35 g).

⑩ MIN Break a sweat

Intersperse your day with three 10-minute fitness hits, such as power walks around the block. (OK, this will take 30 minutes total, but the payoff will be worth it!) You'll burn calories, keep your metabolism humming and get in the general habit of being more active. Only 20 percent of women trying to lose weight say they combine exercise with cutting calories, *The Journal of the American Medical Association* notes, even though those most likely to succeed at slimming down permanently do both.

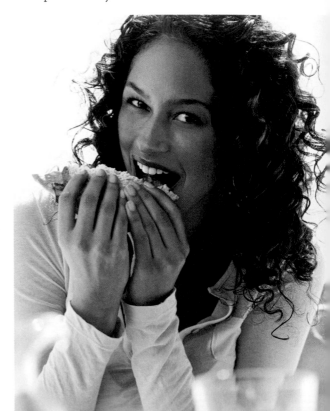

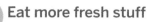

8 MIN Eat more fresh stuff

Make at least one of your daily snacks a piece of fruit or a vegetable and you'll lower your risk of becoming obese. Place fruit and veggies at eye-level in your fridge. Think of it as the see-food diet: You're more likely to eat what's in your line of vision.

10 MIN Diet with a friend

Hook up with a pal and call or e-mail each other when you're tempted to eat something unhealthy. The *Journal of Consulting and Clinical Psychology* reports that dieters who have support from their buddies are more likely to keep the weight off than those who fly solo. Make new diet friends at Self.com.

3 MIN Trim toppings by 50 percent

Use half of your usual amount of regular salad dressing, mayo, butter, syrup, etc. If you're not watching what you pour on or put into your food, you can easily add 500 calories per day without even realizing it. You'll still get plenty of flavor using less.

10 MIN Be a label sleuth

Check the label of foods you eat today for serving sizes. It's easy to be fooled into thinking a packaged product is one serving when it may be two or more. Only 1 percent of Americans surveyed properly identified correct serving sizes for eight different foods, notes the American Institute for Cancer Research in Washington, D.C. Tempted? Split the pack into single servings: one for now; the rest, store in sealable plastic bags.

1 MIN Portion out your plate

Before you serve yourself, mentally divide your dish into quarters: Fill one section with lean protein, such as fish or chicken; one with a healthy carb like brown rice; and the other half with steamed veggies or a green salad. You'll get a balanced proportion of the major food groups without measuring.

15 MIN Close your kitchen at night

Regularly munching after 8 P.M. is linked to weight gain—as much as 1 pound a year. After dinner, stow leftovers, start the dishwasher and flip the light switch to put an end to nibbling. Kitchen closed!

2 MIN Talk to yourself

Before you snack, ask yourself why you want to eat—it might be to soothe anger or stress, not because you're hungry. When you get the urge to indulge, rate your hunger on a scale of 1 to 10, with 1 being ravenous and 10 being stuffed. Grab a snack if you're at 4 or 5. Anything less, find another way to deal with your emotions, like calling a pal.

5 MIN Lighten favorites

Pick lower-calorie, lower-fat versions of the dairy, meats, sodas and snacks you eat often. Many light options are as tasty as the originals and offer an easy way to cut fat and calories while still eating things that make you go *mmm*. For instance, swapping whole milk for skim saves 63 calories and more than 7 g fat per cup. Simple!

1 MIN Cut back on booze

You can easily down an extra 1,000 calories a week with only a few drinks. Plus, drinking lowers your inhibitions, so you might dig into high-fat fare you'd otherwise resist. If you usually have two glasses of wine, drink only one and switch to seltzer or diet soda; or, have one nonalcoholic drink between each alcohol-containing one to control your calorie intake.

1 MIN Give yourself a break

Polished off the bread basket at lunch or ate a pint of ice cream for dinner? Forget about it and get right back on track with your next meal or snack. Expecting to be a flawless eater 100 percent of the time is unreasonable, and feeling guilty about caving in to a craving can cause you to abandon your weight loss efforts. One slip won't make you fat; letting that slip grow into days or weeks of overeating could.

⏱ GOT 15 MINUTES?

Clean up your diet

Need a fresh start to your dieting efforts? Forget detoxing and check out this plan instead: seven days of easy menus that focus on whole, healthy foods to whittle off pounds while removing sugar, fat and processed junk from your body. You can repeat the menus as often as you like, and feel free to mix and match meals. Each day is about 1,500 calories, giving you a sustained energy buzz that will keep you eating right.

DAY 1

DAY 2

DAY 3

BREAKFAST

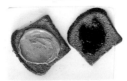

2 slices whole-wheat toast, 1 tbsp all-natural peanut butter on one and 2 tsp all-fruit, low-sugar jam on the other

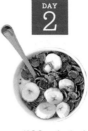

¾ cup (100 calories) lowfat, low-sugar cereal mixed with ½ cup high-fiber cereal, 1 cup skim milk and ½ sliced banana

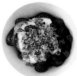

1 cup berries, ¼ cup reduced-fat granola, ½ cup nonfat yogurt mixed with 2 tbsp skim milk

LUNCH

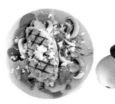

6 oz grilled chicken breast over spinach and mushroom salad, topped with 3 tbsp lowfat dressing and 1 oz feta; 1 pear

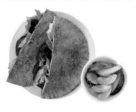

Sandwich: 1 large whole-wheat pita (170 calories) filled with ⅓ cup hummus, shredded arugula, sliced tomatoes and black olives; 1 cup sliced fruit

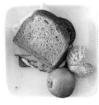

Sandwich: 3 slices turkey, 1 slice lowfat Swiss, 1 tomato slice and 1 tsp lowfat mayo on reduced-calorie whole-wheat bread; 2 clementines

SNACK

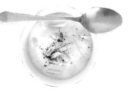

6 oz nonfat vanilla yogurt topped with cinnamon and 2 tbsp slivered almonds

1 oz raw or roasted pecans (20 halves)

1 tbsp all-natural peanut butter with 1 apple or pear

DINNER

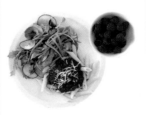

1½ cups cooked pasta, ½ cup tomato sauce (no more than 60 calories), 2 tbsp Parmesan; green salad (all you want), 1 tsp olive oil, splash balsamic vinegar; ¾ cup berries

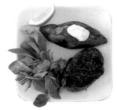

6 oz filet mignon, trimmed of fat; fist-sized baked sweet or regular potato with lemon juice and a small dollop of nonfat sour cream; side salad with 1 tbsp dressing

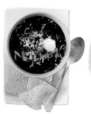

3 cups turkey chili, 1 tbsp onion, 1 tbsp shredded lowfat mozzarella, ¼ cup chopped tomatoes, 1 tsp nonfat sour cream; 10 baked tortilla chips; 1 all-fruit frozen pop

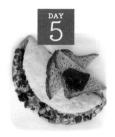

DAY 4

DAY 5

DAY 6

DAY 7

Smoothie: Blend ¾ cup skim milk, 1 frozen banana, 1 cup frozen berries and ¼ cup apple juice

Omelet: 1 whole egg, 3 egg whites, veggies; 1 slice whole-grain toast with 1 tsp all-fruit, low-sugar jam

Toasted oat-bran bagel topped with 2 tsp light cream cheese and 2 oz smoked salmon

Baked apple filled with ½ cup nonfat yogurt and 1½ tbsp walnuts, topped with cinnamon and 2 tsp maple syrup

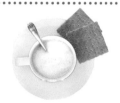

1 veggie burger on a whole-wheat bun with 2 tomato slices, red onion rings, 1 slice lowfat cheese, lettuce leaf and 1 tbsp ketchup; 1 cup fruit salad

Minestrone (300 calories' worth); side salad with 1 tbsp lowfat dressing; ½ oz raisins (small snack box)

Canned light tuna in water (6 oz), 1 tbsp lowfat mayo, 1 tbsp walnuts, 2 tsp dried cranberries; arugula; whole-grain crackers (100 calories)

1 slice thin-crust pizza; side of raw veggies with 2 tbsp lowfat dressing; 1 all-fruit frozen pop (70 calories or fewer)

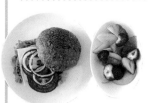
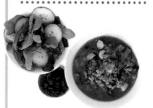
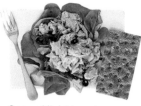
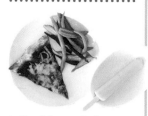

¾ to 1 cup high-fiber cereal, 1 tbsp wheat germ and 1 cup skim milk

1 large skim decaf latte (or 1 cup skim milk); 1 graham cracker sheet

1 small bag soy crisps (1.5 oz) and a wedge (1.5 oz) of lowfat cheese

1 heaping cup fresh fruit salad with a large dollop of nonfat yogurt

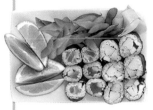
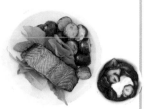
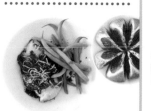
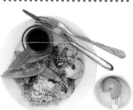

Two 6-piece sushi rolls (any type except tempura, eel or spicy tuna, all of which are higher in calories); 1½ cups unshelled edamame; 1 orange

6 oz broiled wild salmon brushed with mix of 1 tbsp low-sodium soy sauce, 1 tbsp honey; 6 oz roasted red potatoes; arugula; 1 cup berries; 1 tbsp nonfat yogurt

6 oz chicken breast cooked in 1 cup marinara; ½ onion, chopped; garlic; 2 tbsp Parmesan; 1 cup green beans sautéed in 2 tsp olive oil, chopped parsley; 1 grapefruit

Chinese: 1 steamed veggie; ¾ cup steamed shrimp; 1 tbsp garlic or ginger sauce; ¾ cup steamed brown rice; fortune cookie (fortune: "You'll feel great!")

🕐 GOT 8 MINUTES? Become healthier, slimmer, happier

Write down every meal, snack and drink you consume, and how you feel at the time. The payoff: Dieters who logged their intake for eight weeks lost about 4 pounds, while those who didn't gained weight, a study in *Obesity Research* shows. A food diary can help you target times you overdo it, so you can run interference. Photocopy the form here, or keep an online journal by joining the SELF Diet Club (SelfDietClub.com).

DAY & TIME	WHAT I ATE	WHERE I WAS	HOW I FELT

YOUR EAT-RIGHT TO-DON'T LIST

»Don't beat yourself up for any extra pounds. Bashing your body will push you to overeat to soothe your feelings.

»Don't force yourself to eat healthful foods you don't like. Instead, find a tasty substitute with similar nutrients.

»Don't try to diet during the holidays. Research shows you'll probably slim back down on your own once you return to your regular eating habits.

»Don't jump on fad diets. They don't work, period. The weight you shed will come back—plus more.

»Don't banish any food. Everything (even pizza and ice cream!) can fit into a healthy, balanced eating plan.

»Don't ever deprive yourself, or you may end up overeating. If you really crave something, go ahead and eat it!

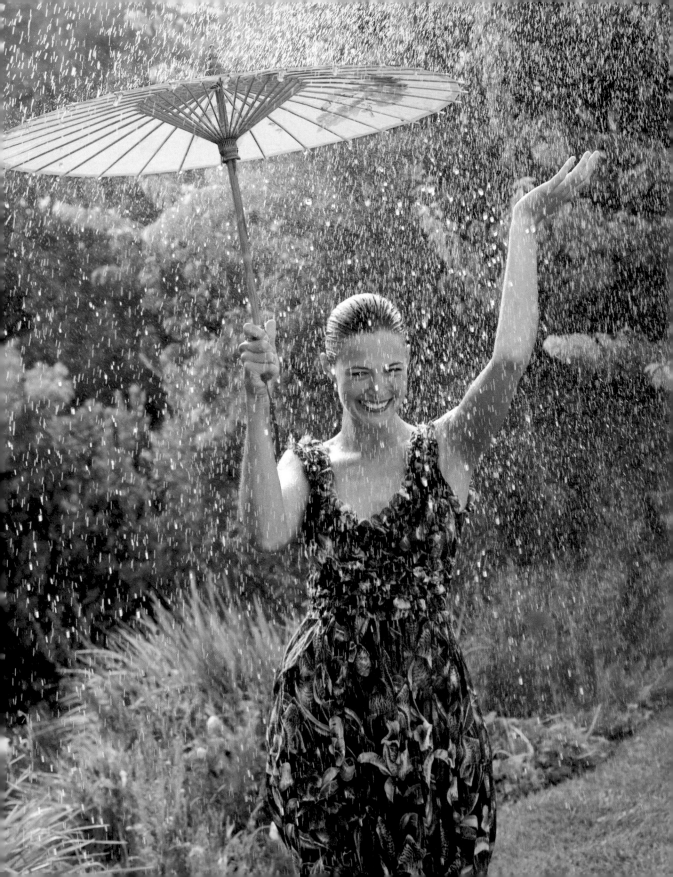

HANDY .
happiness
helpers

Ease your stress, feel more confident
and discover more pleasure in each
and every moment with these tips and
super simple exercises from happiness
experts around the country. If you
spend a few minutes a day practicing the
wisdom that follows, we guarantee your
outlook—as well as your life—will be
more joyful. Get ready to turn "happily
ever after" from fairy tale to reality.

The only 10 things you need to know to feel happier and more fulfilled every day

It's possible to experience more joy right now, whether or not you manage to lose those last 5 pounds, get that hot date or nail that job interview. Deep contentment is less about what you have (or don't have) in life and more about how you *look* at your life and everything in it. Here are 10 proven strategies to help you access, nurture and savor the pleasure you already possess within.

1 Show some appreciation

Romantic love is grand, but there's another kind of love—the kind you feel upon glimpsing a magnificent view after a strenuous hike or spending an afternoon playing with your adorable niece—that may be even more powerful. Better still, this love, which is rooted in appreciation, can blossom without anyone returning it. To flex your gratitude muscle, each night, recall three things that went well for you that day and why. Focus on the good experiences and you'll bask in the warm feelings that accompanied them. Do this for a month and research suggests you'll feel happier—and stay that way even six months later.

2 Go with the flow

There are times when an evening with the remote control is all it takes to feel content. But for lasting fulfillment, you also need to engage in activities that require effort, skill and focus, be it finishing a crossword puzzle or running a marathon. Aim to spend at least 20 percent of your leisure time doing something that gets you into a "flow" state—a frame of mind in which you're fully absorbed and time flies. The satisfaction you'll glean will lift your spirits more than your favorite TV show.

3 Chase your dreams

We all have to work to live (well, most of us do), but it's essential to take regular breaks from the daily grind to do what excites you most. If entertaining is your bag, invite friends for Monday-night Mexican. Love to travel? Research your next trip to Rome. Indulge your passions as often as possible to keep your bliss battery humming along.

4 Pen your own happy ending

Your boss chewed you out. Your best friend is dating your ex. Sure, you feel bad, but it's up to you just how bad. A study from the University

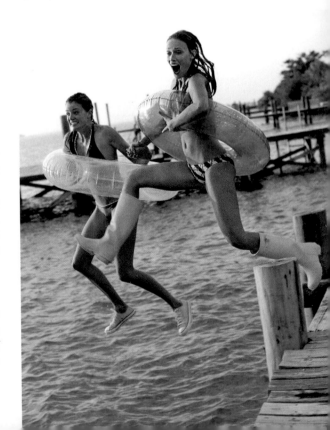

of Michigan at Ann Arbor found that people who brood about a failure are more apt to be depressed six months later than those who let setbacks go. Instead of obsessing over a faux pas, write down your ideal future, starring your best imaginable self. People who put their positive fantasies down on paper reported feeling significantly happier in a month. Be a daydream believer.

5 Walk your talk

Many of us claim to be for something—charity, a cleaner environment—but we don't always find the time or energy to volunteer or recycle those bottles or pick up litter in a local park. As a result, we feel dissatisfied. But align your daily actions with your value system and you'll begin finding joy in the most ordinary moments. If you extol honesty, infuse your daily encounters with integrity to reap well-being. Cherish loyalty? Chat with your best friend weekly to touch base. Practice what you preach and you'll connect to the happiest part of you.

6 Perform random (or not-so-random) acts of kindness

OK, so this is a bumper sticker, but research suggests that doing nice things for others makes you happier, including teeny things like letting a car pull in front of you when everyone is in a rush. Altruistic acts create a circle of virtue: Do something nice for someone and she'll feel grateful and do something nice for you or someone else. Pass the karma on.

7 Remove those blinders

Maybe you want to run a 5K in two months or learn conversational Portuguese before your trip to Brazil: Set a goal (with a deadline), then, instead of obsessing about the end point, focus your attention on the steps that will get you there. True satisfaction doesn't come only at the finish line—much of it lies on the road leading up to it. A caveat: You're likelier to succeed if you frame your aims positively in terms of what you want (e.g., to run a race) rather than what you don't want (e.g., those extra 5 pounds).

8 Come together

A knitting circle, a running club and a local church are more than merely good places to meet and mingle. Pursuing noble causes—such as friendship, spiritual growth, art or learning—helps you find meaning in life and gives you hope, which ultimately translates to a happier you. Studies show that joining a gathering of people who've convened for a common cause focused on the greater good, such as a conservation club or an adult education class, is as beneficial to your health as quitting smoking or exercising on a regular basis. So find some like-minded souls and start making connections!

9 Apply your strengths

People tend to be happiest when they're doing what they're best at. The trouble is, not everything we do requires our enviable talents. It is possible, however, to channel your aptitudes into your day-to-day tasks. First, identify five of your strongest traits (e.g., intelligence, kindness, humor). Then reflect on ways you can hone your gifts in your ordinary routine. If your strength is community building and you're in sales, for instance, try viewing cold calls as a way of reaching out to others. You'll discover inspiration and motivation in the most mundane tasks.

10 Make your happy heart pound

There are dozens of physical benefits to exercise, but the most profound perk might be the zip it gives your mood. Research indicates that only three brief workouts a week can improve your outlook nearly as well as antidepressants. "Rarely in science do we say yes so definitively to any question, but does exercise boost mood? Absolutely," says Marie-Annette Brown, Ph.D., a professor in the School of Nursing at the University of Washington in Seattle. Exercise increases blood flow and produces more feel-good serotonin. "It also improves alertness and alleviates fatigue, irritability, anxiety and carbohydrate cravings," Brown says. You'll be smiling nonstop.

◔ GOT 5 MINUTES? Let your troubles go

Sometimes, all it takes to turn your weaknesses into roaring strengths is a minor tweak in perspective. Here's what you can do to make that happen.

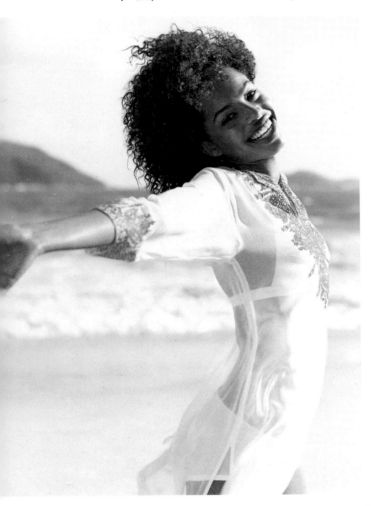

Afraid to speak up? Teach yourself to be more assertive by using your imagination. The next time you're feeling tongue-tied, think of your most self-confident, outspoken friend. How would she act in the situation? Model your next move on her.

Losing patience? Stop fuming over the fact that your waiter is ignoring you and focus on five positive things around you—e.g., the sun streaming through a window or the rich sound of a good friend's laughter. Distract yourself and you'll be better able to savor the present rather than rushing through it.

Acting like a grouch? It's not so hard to conjure some cheer if you put a bit of thought into it. Make a point of answering the phone with a "Good morning!" Greet the receptionist when you get to work. Soon, sunniness will be second nature.

Scared the sky will fall? The more you give in to fear, the more it rules you. So dare yourself to do things that intimidate you, such as eating in a restaurant solo, and you'll find that the more you take risks, the more you'll be willing to take.

Down on everyone? No one loves a critic. Tell your friends to remind you when you're being negative. Then replace nay-saying with sincere compliments. Repeat until it becomes habit.

Always fretting? Think about what's behind your angst. Your worry (maybe this freckle is cancer!) could be masking a solvable problem (you should take better care of yourself). Seeing that there is no reason for jitters makes it easier to release them.

◔ GOT 10 MINUTES?
Break a habit

Venturing out of your comfort zone can trigger the release of dopamine, a mood-lifting neurotransmitter, and leave you feeling fab. Draw up a numbered list of six things you want to try (biking to work). Roll one die a day and try the number that comes up. You can't lose!

⏱ GOT 2 MINUTES?
Start the day right

Before you hit the sheets, set your alarm two minutes earlier than usual. When you wake, resist the urge to press SNOOZE and use the time to reflect on things you're thankful for. Studies show that practicing grateful thinking makes people more energetic and enthusiastic. You won't miss the 120 seconds of sleep, we promise!

⏱ GOT 10 MINUTES?
Shake off a blue mood

Research shows that two of the best ways to lift your spirits are exercise and music, so pump up the jams and dance around; you'll shift into high-energy mode. Check out SELF's cardio mixes at Self.com/go/music.

⏱ GOT 4 MINUTES?
Banish the negative

Become a glass-is-half-full person with this uplifting tip from Randy Larsen, Ph.D., psychology professor at Washington University in St. Louis. Spend two minutes "horriblizing" any situation ("I'm giving a speech and I'll bomb!"). Then take two to "possiblize" it ("I'll kick butt and get a raise!"). Which way would you rather think—and live?

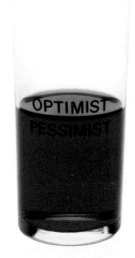

⏱ GOT 9 MINUTES?
Look to the future
Want to be happier with your lot? Grab a pen and try the steps below to make peace with your mistakes.

1 **WRITE DOWN A PAST DECISION** that makes you cringe. Perhaps you stayed too long in a dead-end job or dated the wrong guy against everyone's advice.

2 **GIVE YOURSELF CREDIT** rather than putting the gaffe out of your mind. Instead of wondering what might have been, which will only fuel discontent, record the fact that you've gotten through the ordeal and have learned something in the process. Use that newfound strength to move forward.

3 **CULTIVATE COMPASSION** for the old you and call a moratorium on negative self-talk: Don't berate yourself for a "bad" move; strive to understand what informed your choice. Maybe you didn't realize you could change positions in your company, or perhaps you simply needed the job to pay bills. This perspective will make it easier for you to stop judging yourself.

4 **PUT YOUR PERSONAL HISTORY INTO CONTEXT** by looking at a disappointing event as one instance in a series of events that make up your life. Note what you've learned from it and how it has changed your relationships. ("I met my best pal at that lame job.") Smart or not, your choices have undoubtedly led to new people and passions you wouldn't have gained otherwise. So jettison those regrets once and for all!

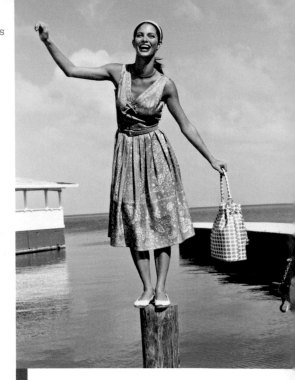

⏲ GOT 5 MINUTES?
Master the art of idling

A STUDY in the *Journal of Marriage and Family* found that women tend to feel rushed regardless of how much time we have to ourselves. "Rather than relishing a break, we're tyrannized by thoughts of what we *should* do," explains Larina Kase, Psy.D., a psychologist in Philadelphia. We book up our free time and never allow ourselves those necessary quiet lulls that replenish our energy. So stop. Breathe. And try these suggestions for savoring your stolen moments.

START SMALL Practice being alone and quiet in small increments to get more comfortable with it. Instead of grabbing your cell while in line at the ATM, let your mind wander. Use the pause to reflect.

AVOID JUGGLING Multitasking may be a boon at the office, but it can become a bad habit when you're off the clock. "Checking voice mail while watching CNN and reading the Sunday paper can diffuse your attention and leave you feeling frazzled," Kase says. Luxuriate in doing a single activity such as browsing through a favorite cookbook for new recipes.

DREAM A LITTLE DREAM Never mind what you think you need to be doing or what your friends are doing. Contemplate your ideal way to spend an evening or weekend. Longing to surf the Web for new furniture? Rent a mindless chick flick? Play Sudoku for two hours straight? Once you've identified your favorite ways to spend your free moments, you're bound to crave more of them.

GOT 30 SECONDS?
Just say no
Repeat this: "Thanks, but I can't take that on right now." If your plate is too full, don't commit to more. Then congratulate yourself on setting healthy limits.

⏲ GOT 2 MINUTES?
Achieve balance

Sometimes it's tough to keep your job from overlapping with your personal life, but "integrating the two can waste time," says Ellen Kossek, Ph.D., professor of organizational behavior at Michigan State University in East Lansing. "It takes extra energy to do two things at once." To find out if you're an integrator (you merge work and home) or a separator (you don't if you can help it), check those that apply:

☐ I use one calendar for work and family.

☐ I take calls from the office after hours.

☐ I do personal tasks during the workday.

☐ I check work e-mail on weekends.

☐ My kitchen table is also my home office.

If you marked three or more, you're an integrator. To control your tendency to merge, spend two minutes each morning plotting your work and home priorities and allotting a contained block of time to accomplish each. You can still run errands between 9 and 5, but when your time is up, resolve to switch gears and focus.

🕐 GOT 6 MINUTES?

Beat Sunday-night blues
There's a reason no one says, "Thank God it's Sunday!" A Self.com poll finds that 63 percent of women view it as a gloomy day, when looming work responsibilities move to the fore. Fight the doldrums with these weekend-enhancing strategies.

Sunday bummer	Sunday booster
All good things must end. The fun part of the week is over; now there's nothing left to think of but work!	**Don't let socializing end with the weekend.** Schedule a low-key dinner with a favorite pal on Sunday evening to take the sting out of the fact that tomorrow is Monday. And make a point of planning movie dates or dinners with friends during the week so you have something to look forward to.
Your to do list is endless. Sunday means buying groceries, paying bills, doing laundry, ironing, scrubbing the bathtub. Fun, huh?	**Be creative with scheduling.** Separate your errands into must-dos and can-waits by asking yourself what's the worst that would happen if you didn't get to a certain job. If you're out of clean undies, then laundry is a must, but do you really need to iron every last wrinkled thing in your closet? Pepper your tasks throughout the week so Sunday is less of a slog.
You have office anxiety. Sunday nights remind you of all the fires you have to put out when you get to your desk in the morning.	**Nip stress in the bud.** Spend a few minutes thinking about possible solutions to tomorrow's problems. Then leave yourself a voice mail at work detailing the issue (a stalled project) and the proposed solution (a brainstorming meeting). Devising concrete solutions will help clear your mind so you can enjoy what's left of your weekend, not to mention sleep soundly.

🕐 GOT 4 MINUTES?
Plan a road trip

For low-stress driving, ask yourself these questions before you set out:
● Where to go? See RoadsideAmerica .com for quirky holiday destinations that aren't overrun with tourists.
● When to go? Search for road-construction snafus at RandMcNally.com. To learn about delays in 40 cities, call 866-MY-TRAFC.
● What's the cost? Find out with AAA's FuelCostCalculator.com. Simply select your starting city, destination and car's make.

🕐 GOT 8 MINUTES?
Unplug yourself

Can't resist looking at your office e-mail even when you're supposed to be off duty? Give in to that inner worker bee, but only in moderation. Log on once a night for peace of mind, then stick an off-limits Post-it on your computer. (Oh, and be sure to obey it!)

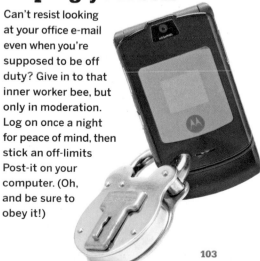

🕙 GOT 10 MINUTES? Uncover your brilliance

The more aware you are of your native strengths, the more you'll use them to their fullest. Check the statements that best describe you to gain self-insight. (Ignore the abbreviations that follow each; we will tell you what they mean at the end.)

☐ I'd rather draw a map than give someone verbal directions. (S)

☐ I play a musical instrument (or I used to play one). (M)

☐ I link music with my moods. (M)

☐ I do calculations in my head. (LM)

☐ I like working with calculators. (LM)

☐ I pick up dance steps quickly. (BK)

☐ I can express myself easily. (L)

☐ I enjoy hearing a good lecture or speech. (L)

☐ I'm always able to tell north from south. (S)

☐ Life would seem empty without music. (M)

☐ I can follow the directions that come with new gadgets. (S)

☐ I like puzzles and games. (S)

☐ Learning to ride a bike was easy for me. (BK)

☐ Illogical statements bug me. (LM)

☐ I'm well coordinated. (BK)

☐ I see number patterns easily. (LM)

☐ I like working with my hands. (BK)

☐ I'm good at discerning the fine points of word meanings. (L)

☐ I can look at an object and easily envision how it would look sideways or backward. (S)

☐ I often connect a song with some event or time in my life. (M)

☐ I like looking at the shapes of buildings and structures. (S)

☐ I like working with numbers. (LM)

☐ I hum or sing when alone. (M)

☐ I'm good at sports. (BK)

☐ I'm interested in language. (L)

☐ I'm usually aware of the expression on my face. (INTRA)

☐ I'm sensitive to the expressions on other people's faces. (INTER)

☐ I'm aware of my moods. (INTRA)

☐ I am generally aware of other people's moods. (INTER)

☐ I can usually get a good sense of what other people think of me. (INTRA)

SCORING L stands for linguistic ability; LM for logic/mathematics; M for musical abilities. S stands for spatial intelligence, which is strong in people with good visual skills; BK for bodily-kinesthetic intelligence, pronounced in athletes and dancers. INTER stands for interpersonal skills and INTRA for intrapersonal intelligence (self-awareness), often found in psychologists and writers. Checking four letters from the same category in the first 25 statements means you have a strong ability in that area; one or more checks per category in the last 5 statements suggests a bent for those traits. Bored at work? Think about whether what you do plays to your strengths. If not, flex your mental muscles in a new gig, or add more stimulating after-work pursuits to your daily life.

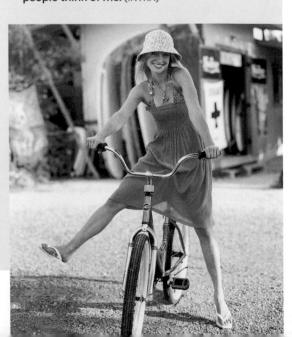

🕐 GOT 10 MINUTES?
Spark your creativity
Induce more *aha* moments with these exercises.

MAKE A WONDER LIST Jot down 10 experiences that have made an impact on you, whether riding a hot-air balloon or listening to a favorite writer read. Thinking about something inspiring will get your ideas flowing.

TAKE A LONG BATH Ever notice how the strongest ideas come to you when you're in the bathtub or on the treadmill or doing just about anything but thinking about being creative? Sometimes, the best ideas come unbidden.

PAY ATTENTION When insight strikes unexpectedly (for instance, when you're soaking), record your idea, along with where you were and what you were doing, to clue you in to when you do your best thinking. Genius!

🕐 GOT 3 MINUTES?
Enhance your brainpower

Chomp on a piece of gum. People who chewed for three minutes before and during memory tests bested nonchewers by 35 percent, a study from the University of Northumbria in England finds. It seems gum lovers' hearts pumped faster, bringing more oxygen and insulin to the brain.

🕐 GOT 8 MINUTES?
Wake up your mind

Channel autumn's back-to-school vibe any time of the year by getting a little education: Check out your alma mater's English department courses online and rediscover a literary classic. Or attend an Ivy, albeit virtually, by logging on to Princeton University (English.Princeton.edu). Review the course options; if a class catches your eye, choose an author or take on the entire reading list. Then make like a student by burying yourself in a book—this time, you get an A for merely doing your homework.

🕐 GOT 3 MINUTES?
Improve your memory

MOST PEOPLE remember things using either visual cues or verbal ones. By figuring out which you typically gravitate toward, you can learn to store memories in the dominant part of your brain and hold on to them longer.

When I am driving somewhere I've never been, it is generally easier for me to...
a. Navigate using landmarks.   b. Follow street signs.

If I'm doodling, I tend to...
a. Draw pictures.   b. Write words.

When I have free time, I'd rather...
a. Watch TV.   b. Listen to the radio.

MOSTLY As? You're a picture person. Should you want to store something on your internal hard drive, convert verbal data to visual. For instance, when you remove your shoes, pause to take a mental snapshot of where they are.

MOSTLY Bs? You're a words woman. When you get visual information, attach a verbal cue to it. If you see your shoes on the floor, for example, say to yourself, "My shoes are next to the coffee table." The memory trick will be useful when you're rushing to get dressed for work.

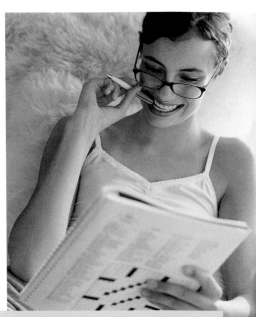

⏱ GOT 3 MINUTES?
Analyze your downtime

News flash: Not every so-called time-wasting activity is actually a waste of your precious minutes. Research suggests that controlled dallying, done before tackling must-do chores, can actually be good for you. Chronic, put-everything-off procrastination, on the other hand, has been shown to lead to anxiety and even depression. So stop worrying about what you *should* be doing (it's OK, really!) and use these clues to see if your dawdling habits are fruitful or futile.

You're a healthy dawdler if	You're an unhealthy dawdler if
You set time-wasting parameters. That means deciding beforehand how long you'll watch TV (as opposed to vegging out on the sofa for hours on end) and then sticking to the limit you've imposed. (Set a timer if you have to.) Not only will you be more productive, but you'll also be less likely to go to bed wondering, Where did the day go?	**You tend to save huge projects for the last minute.** Better to procrastinate (and accomplish) in stages. If you're hosting a bash in three weeks, send a save-the-date e-mail, then worry about the menu the next week. When that time comes, ponder food and drink, then make a list. You'll satisfy the need to put off while inching toward your goal.
You diverge creatively. Give yourself brownie points for penning a poem to delay writing a report; being creative in any way gets the juices flowing. Better yet, engage in a task that's relevant to the project at hand, such as snapping family pics instead of composing your parents' anniversary toast.	**You invite distraction.** When your e-mail is chiming, your phone is ringing and the radio is blaring, you're setting yourself up for projectus interruptus. Banish the background noise to sharpen your focus. Unplug, press MUTE, hit the OFF button. Then savor the silence and let your thoughts flow forth!

⏱ GOT 5 MINUTES?
Hold a stress rehearsal

Got performance anxiety? When you're practicing your moves (a speech you're giving for work), get your heart racing by running up stairs or doing jumping jacks. When you're before an audience, the shakiness won't throw you.

⏱ GOT 1 MINUTE?
Relax in the office

Hunching over a keyboard makes arms tense. Send your body a "loosen up" signal with this stretch: Extend your arms forward at chest level, rotating your right arm to the left (so your palm faces out). Use your left hand to bend right fingers back. Hold for 10 seconds. Switch hands; repeat.

⊕ GOT 1 MINUTE?
Show off those pearly whites

Feeling frazzled? Bring on a smile by holding a pen between your teeth, which actually tricks your brain into grinning mode so you *feel* happier and, we hope, more relaxed. Three cheers for faking it!

⊕ GOT 10 MINUTES?
Adopt a mantra

When your thoughts are racing, pick a word you're neutral about (*peace*), and breathe deeply for 10 minutes, repeating it on exhales. Feel better fast.

⊕ GOT 8 MINUTES?
Give yourself a reality check

Some stress can make you more productive. Too much stress will sap your enjoyment of life. To help you find equilibrium, write down everything that's causing you angst, rational or not. Next, decide which things are unavoidable (getting to work on time) and which are mostly self-imposed (cooking dinner every night). Then drop as many of the latter as possible. After all, does feeding your family a healthy take-out dinner (or asking your partner to do it) make you a bad person? Nope.

⊕ GOT 5 MINUTES?
Rub your head

Maybe a week at a spa isn't in your budget. But you can still take your stress into your own hands, literally, with this simple massage technique from the Hôtel Guanahani and Spa in St. Bart's.

1 **SIT IN A QUIET PLACE** Bend your head and rest your eyes in the palm of your hands. Breathe in and out through your nose, slowly and deeply, for about one minute.

2 **RAISE YOUR HEAD** Keeping your eyes closed, place yours palm on your temples, with your fingers on your crown. Push firmly inward for 20 seconds or so.

3 **SLIDE YOUR HANDS BACK** Pressing palms into temples, move hands in a circular motion, so your scalp moves beneath, for one minute. Repeat entire sequence.

GOT 30 SECONDS?
Sigh away stress

Try this relaxer from the Mayflower Spa in Washington, Connecticut: Inhale deeply. Exhale loudly and imagine worries streaming out with the sound.

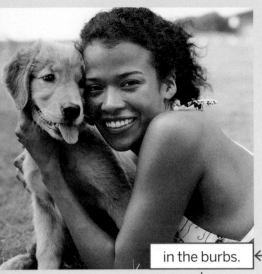

🕐 GOT 3 MINUTES?

Find your ideal Fido

Having a pooch around can make you happier, reduce anxiety and even improve your health and sense of well-being long-term. Use this flowchart to help ensure you end up with the pick of the litter.

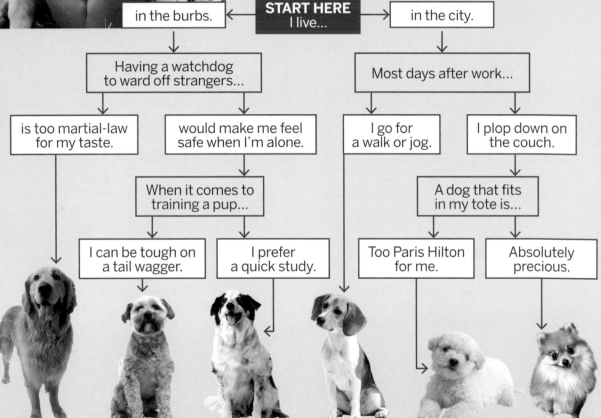

in the burbs. ← **START HERE** I live... → in the city.

Having a watchdog to ward off strangers...

Most days after work...

is too martial-law for my taste.

would make me feel safe when I'm alone.

I go for a walk or jog.

I plop down on the couch.

When it comes to training a pup...

A dog that fits in my tote is...

I can be tough on a tail wagger.

I prefer a quick study.

Too Paris Hilton for me.

Absolutely precious.

SPORTING
Friendly golden retrievers are the darling of this group. But they shed profusely. Spaniels are a less hairy option.

TERRIER
Playful and alert, these scrappy dogs, like the Wheaton, bark at strangers and may be destructive unless trained.

HERDING
Easy to train but territorial, breeds like border collies and German shepherds were bred to keep flocks together.

HOUNDS
Smaller-sized hounds such as a beagle, whippet or basenji can be good workout buddies and enjoy apartment living.

NONSPORTING
For a compact pooch that will be content to go for short daily walks, consider the French bulldog or check out a bichon frise.

TOYS
These petite pets can be mellow, like a pug, or feisty, like a Pomeranian. Note: Tiny toys may be too fragile if you have kids.

🕐 GOT 6 MINUTES?
Unwind anywhere!

TRY THESE LENGTHENING stretches from tai chi expert Scott Cole, in Palm Springs, California:

BENDING BEAR Stand with feet slightly apart and turned out, knees soft. Exhale, bend forward and let head and hands hang. Inhale; slowly round up. Turn torso to left; repeat, lowering to left. Repeat to right, then repeat entire sequence.
DAN TIEN CONNECTION Stand with feet slightly apart. Rounding arms, bring fingertips together (almost touching) at hip level, palms up. Inhale; draw hands up, bending elbows. As hands reach chest level, turn wrists in so palms are down. Exhale, relaxing arms to start. Do five times.

🕐 GOT 2 MINUTES?
Feel in control at work

Quell job jitters with this tip: Close your eyes and take five breaths. Think of the task ahead and a talent of yours (creativity) that will be key to the project. Envision it finished. Soon, it will be!

🕐 GOT 5 MINUTES?
Shower away tension

Try this wake-up call from Barbara Ann Kipfer, Ph.D.,of Essex, Connecticut: Let the water beat on your head; take three breaths; focus on sensations; pretend you're washing off angst. Close your eyes and say, "I'm refreshed," savoring the serenity.

🕐 GOT 8 MINUTES?
Take the pressure off

One of the keys to living a happier life is having fewer expectations—and that doesn't mean lowering your standards. Learn to be less outcome-obsessed with this exercise from psychologist Susan Jeffers of Los Angeles.

1 On a sheet of paper, list your top 20 hopes for the future.
Example "I hope I will get married. I hope I'll get that job in television writing. I hope to lose 20 pounds before my college reunion."

2 Now substitute the words *wonder if* for *hope,* and then rewrite the phrases again.
Example "I wonder if I'll get married? I wonder if I'll get that job in television? I wonder if I'll lose 20 pounds before my college reunion?"

3 Reflect on whether your emotions differ when you write *I wonder if* versus *I hope.*
What you may feel Relieved. "Letting go can ease the pressure. It helps you learn to enjoy the journey, not only the goal," Jeffers says.

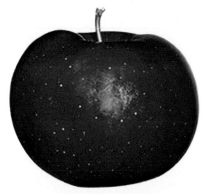

🕐 GOT 1 MINUTE?
Soothe morning moods

Beat A.M. tension with therapeutic sniffing: Instead of a cup of java, have cider or vanilla chai tea. "Apple and vanilla scents increase the brain's calming alpha waves," says Alan Hirsch, M.D., neurological director of the Smell & Taste Treatment and Research Foundation in Chicago.

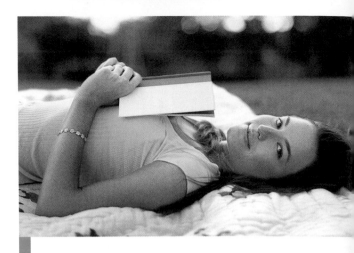

⏱ GOT 5 MINUTES?
Figure out if you're an approval addict

CARING TOO MUCH about others' opinions can be a sign your confidence needs a lift. Take this quickie quiz to find out the state of your ego.

1 Which description best matches you?
a I'm selfless; I put others' needs first.
b I'm timid; I rarely take the spotlight.
c I'm a straight shooter; I say what I mean.
d I'm laid-back; I take life as it comes.

2 You're offered your dream job—across the country. Before deciding, how many people do you consult? _____

3 Your new man is 15 years your senior. People say, "Too old!" You say: _____

Assess your answers
1 If you said A or B, you might be an approval hound. Stop asking, "What do you want?" and ask, "What do *I* want?" Quiet types should practice offering opinions with pals. Most likely they'll respect your input, which will help you gain courage to express yourself more often.
2 If you solicited feedback from half of your circle, it's a sign you don't trust your instincts. If you find you're ignoring advice that doesn't jibe with what you already think, stop polling.
3 If you said anything but "Thanks—it works for me," then you put too much stock in others' opinions. Discuss the relationship with someone who knows you; the gal in yoga class who says older guys are bad in bed doesn't count.

⏱ GOT 5 MINUTES?
Attain body confidence
Try out these ego-friendly options.

INSTEAD OF THIS	DO THIS
Heading straight for the self-help aisle and snatching up the latest fad diet or exercise book du jour every time you step into a bookstore…	**Make a beeline for a page-turner** or a riveting biography of a woman you admire. Then ask yourself if anyone cared about this woman's dress size.
Stepping on the bathroom scale every morning and letting the number dictate your mood and how you feel about yourself all day…	**Create a new morning ritual** such as taking five minutes to scan your datebook to remind yourself of an event you're looking forward to.
Taping a photograph of your favorite celebrity waif on your refrigerator to ward off ice cream cravings and stealth potato chip sessions…	**Display a photograph of yourself** outside doing a favorite activity with your friends or playing with your kids and remind yourself of your rich life!

⏱ GOT 6 MINUTES?
Channel good vibes

Watching TV for a few minutes may bolster your self-esteem, researchers at the University of Pennsylvania in Philadelphia say. Students given poor results on a fake IQ test felt better about themselves after tuning in for only six minutes, regardless of what they viewed. Hate the tube? Scientists say any distracting activity can work in much the same way.

⏱ GOT 15 MINUTES?

Play bod libs! What would life be like if you loved your body? Ask a good friend to read the prompts beneath the blanks out loud, and record your answers. Peruse the results. Laugh your patootie off.

If I woke up one morning suddenly adoring my body, the first thing I'd do is

_____ . I'd allow myself to eat _____ when I felt like it without any
act you long to do   favorite treat

_____ because I'd know that moderation, not deprivation, is the healthiest
negative emotion

way to go. I'd exercise to have fun and feel good (rather than primarily to work

off last night's dessert), so I'd stop _____ and _____ instead. At work, I'd
                                        dreaded exercise   favorite exercise

finally be fearless enough to ask my boss for _____ , and I'd probably get it,
                                               goal at work

too. But if I didn't, I know it would simply be because my boss is a(n) _____ .
                                                                        insulting name

When I got home from the office, a romp between the sheets would be

_____ because I wouldn't be bashful about ripping off my clothes. Hell, I bet
glowing adjective

it would be better than that scene in _____ . Afterward, I'd burn my
                                      steamy movie

_____ and wear _____ and _____ to _____ , to _____'s
your "fat day" outfit   your feel-sexy outfit   favorite sexy shoes   favorite nightspot   person in the room

house and even to do _____ without a shred of self-consciousness. Or I'd go
                     weekend errand

out to a party and spend more energy _____ and less trying to resist
                                      action verb (with -ing)

the siren call of the _____ or clinging to the wall feeling insecure. I might
                      party food

even _____ . In fact, if I focused more on my body's awe-inspiring ability to
     brazen action

_____ rather than on how I look, I'd probably start calling myself _____ .
physical achievement   female superhero

Plus, with all the money I'd save not buying _____ , I'd have extra cash to put
                                             dumb diet purchase

toward _____ . One thing is for sure: I wouldn't give a hoot if my _____
       dream in need of $$ body part(s)

was/were starting to sag because I'd be too busy toasting my _____ .
                                                            personal strength

⏱ GOT 15 MINUTES?

Leave the office quicker We've pinpointed five major work time wasters along with tips to tackle them so you'll be flush with extra hours for you, you, you!

Master meeting mania

Meetings are the ultimate time-suck. Tame the endless powwow by avoiding long stories and speaking in bullet points. No one needs to know the entire background of how you and Cindi decided to up the budget. Say, "Cindi and I think we need to increase our budget; we've asked Bill to crunch some numbers." If you tend to be a gabber, make a brief, relevant counterpoint after someone speaks rather than rushing to jump in first. Or employ drastic means to keep meetings short: Hold them standing up for maximum discomfort.

Quit phone tag

Learn to use old-fashioned voice communication to your benefit. Rather than responding to each ring, let voice mail pick up for a set period, say, 9 A.M. to 11 A.M., then return calls in batches. If you need to talk to a person rather than leave a message, do it close to 9 A.M. or 5 P.M.; people are more apt to be in and not as crazed as during the midday rush. On your outgoing message, ask people to leave their number first so you don't have to listen to five minutes of rambling.

Clear your space

Think of your desk as the cockpit of a plane—there's a limited surface so you want to use it wisely, primarily for working but also for storing the tools and information you use most often. "I tell people to examine everything on their desk to see if it deserves to be there," says Lisa Zaslow, founder of Gotham Organizers in New York City. Winnow down to the essentials: your computer, Rolodex, day planner, to do list, notepad, pens that work. Ditch the rest. You'll not only make progress faster but more comfortably.

Knock out interruptions

Taking a watercooler-schmoozing break can foster creativity and recharge your brain, but the recess should be planned and for a finite time period. Block off 15-minute slots for visiting with colleagues; beyond that, limit chatting to when you're walking through the office. When you're in your office, shut the door and log off of instant messaging. You'll be more efficient and make time for after-work socializing.

Hit delete

"Checking e-mail is the biggest obsessive-compulsive disorder I've seen," says Laura Stack, a productivity coach in Highlands Ranch, Colorado. "People hear the chime and feel an uncontrollable urge to look." Reality is, only about 1 in 10 messages is important. First, use a junk filter to get rid of the penis-enlargement offers. Then limit checking to once an hour; that is often enough to catch key messages. Make everyone else's life easier by using precise subject-line headers—"Staff meeting rescheduled for 4 P.M."—and include "Needs no reply." You'll dispatch messages with, well, dispatch!

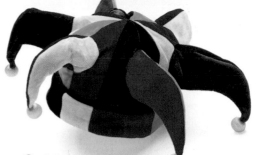

🕐 GOT 10 MINUTES?
Be your own talent scout

Want to live your dream life? Let your skills, passions and instincts show you how.

1 List all the activities you do easily (whatever seems nearly effortless or whatever you know you do better than most people). They could be anything, including helping friends get through emotional crises and programming TiVo.

2 Note the activities in which you are able to lose yourself (in other words, time seems to fly by when you do them), including hobbies and physical chores.

3 List all the activities that make you happy, including the ones you do solely for yourself, with no promise of gain, simply because you find them to be enjoyable, interesting and fulfilling.

4 Compare the three lists to find the overlap: They are likely to be your areas of natural aptitude and talent, where your greatest potential lies. Seek out career and volunteer opportunities that will help you do the things you love most and are best at; you'll spend more time in the happy zone.

🕐 GOT 3 MINUTES?
Remember your password

So many passwords, so little memory. Computer pro Mark Burnett, author of *Perfect Passwords* (Syngress), who has analyzed more than 2 million of them, suggests distinctive (that is, funny!) and hard to crack codes.

Write longer passwords. Phrases ("RollerskateIsGreat") are easier to recall and tougher for hackers to figure out than any single word.

Borrow catchy lyrics. Use a song title ("HotelCalifornia") or a favorite quotation ("LetThemEatCake").

Create a fake e-mail address. Try something like grneggs@seuss.com.

GOT 30 SECONDS?
Find the sweet spot

Each of us has a daily window when we're fresh. To ID yours, think of when you're usually alert yet calm. Do key tasks then to blaze through the day.

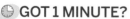

🕐 GOT 1 MINUTE?
Ensure you're paid what you're worth

Curious to know how your earnings stack up? Quick—go to Salary.com to get a look at what peers in your field are making. If your annual compensation is below par for what you're doing and where you live, it might be time for a chat with your boss.

🕐 GOT 10 MINUTES?
Find out if you're happy at work

Take this test to see if a subpar work situation is sabotaging your success.

1 You typically spend ___ hours of your workday stealing mini-breathers.

2 Your boss is sending you to a three-day time-management seminar. You feel...

a Resentful. You're doing fine, thanks very much.
b Excited. Tips *and* you'll get a break from routine? *Yes!*
c Resigned. You're swamped, but maybe this could help.
d Panic. Missing work will sink you for sure.

3 Your definition of socializing at work is...

a Chatting about business matters, period.
b Sharing the latest hot gossip at the coffee machine.
c After-hours get-togethers at the local bar.
d Checking in with a friendly coworker twice a day or so.

4 Rate your relationship with your boss on an average day on a scale of 1 to 5 (5 being excellent, 1 being I'd better keep my head down or she may notice me). ___

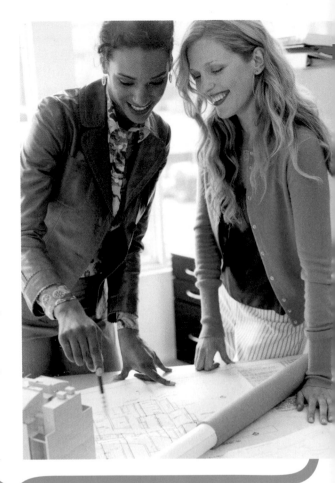

Check your happiness quotient

1 YOU LOVE YOUR JOB IF YOU ANSWERED THAT YOU SPEND AN HOUR AND A HALF OR LESS ON BREAKS
It's reasonable to reserve a portion of your day for meeting your own needs, but if you're ducking out on duties for a good chunk of the day, you may be avoiding something or be stuck in a rut. Ask yourself why you're procrastinating: Are you dreading a difficult project, or do you need to clear your head? Recognizing your motives is the first step to being happier on the job.

2. YOU LOVE YOUR JOB IF YOU ANSWERED B
If you have no time and/or no desire to improve your skills or shake up your routine, you're probably not fully engaged. After all, people who are continually learning are nearly immune to career boredom.

3 YOU LOVE YOUR JOB IF YOU ANSWERED C OR D
Regular, healthy socializing with colleagues can make the difference between liking what you do and loving it. So go ahead and forge those bonds; having a true friend or two at the office can help keep you motivated over the long haul. But don't let the socializing devolve into a nonstop office-gossip fest.

4 YOU LOVE YOUR JOB IF YOU ANSWERED 4 OR 5
A shaky relationship with your boss can spoil any job. To improve interactions, make a list of things you can try to build better rapport. Then invite your manager to lunch to see what makes her tick. Ditch your defensiveness and ask how you can be more effective at what you do. If you can improve the way you react to your boss, chances are, you'll work better together.

GOT 1 MINUTE?
Learn when to say yes to a pay cut

Making a lateral or a downward move, moneywise, isn't always a negative thing. Find out when less dough is the way to go.

SAY YES TO LESS IF

You're unemployed or shifting careers.	But be sure that your new, lower paycheck falls within the industry average for what you'll be doing.
Your stress level will dip.	When a position offers flexible or fewer hours (more vacation or a friendlier environment), moving on could be healthier for you, especially if the rest of your life usually feels crazed.
Fresh learning opportunities are in store.	New duties can jolt your career. Be certain, though, that you will be given challenges and not merely a puffed-up title. Future bosses will care more about what you did, not what you were called.

GOT 2 MINUTES?
Turn sobs into smiles

IF THINGS GET emotional at work, keep your cool by trying these techniques:

APPLY PRESSURE Poking your finger with the end of a paper clip will shift your focus, activating the part of the brain that controls impulse, notes Larina Kase, Psy.D., a psychologist in Philadelphia. More self-control will equal fewer tears.

JUT OUT YOUR JAW "As soon as your eyes well up, push your jaw forward in an underbite," Kase suggests. Apparently, it's difficult to sob and make a silly face at the same time.

GO FOR A QUICK WALK Removing yourself restores calm, and being active stimulates feel-good endorphins that help counter a weepy mood. And if you still cry, at least you're out of sight.

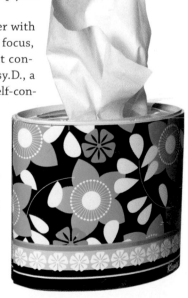

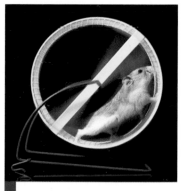

GOT 5 MINUTES?
Get cracking!

It might not be laziness that makes you spin your wheels. It could be fear—of failure or success, experts say. If procrastinating has become a problem, try these tips.

1 Adjust your expectations. Your work doesn't have to be perfect, just good enough.

2 ID the most critical steps, then plan to spend 80 percent of your time on them. When you narrow your focus, it's easier to jump right in.

3 If you think fear of success is blocking you, ask yourself if you'd rather deal with envy or job stagnation.

GOT 4 MINUTES?
Enjoy a chuckle

Facing an intractable problem at the office? Schedule lunch with someone who makes you giggle. Volunteers who watched a funny video for 15 minutes felt twice as hopeful as people who viewed a neutral clip, according to one study. We can't guarantee you'll find your fix, but you're likely to tackle it more optimistically.

🕐 GOT 15 MINUTES?

Effect a lasting change When it comes
to transforming your life (in big or little ways), a bit of
preparation can make all the difference. So instead
of vaguely vowing to be healthier or lose weight, use
this fun exercise to zero in on exactly what you
need to do to vanquish a bad habit or two or achieve
a long-dreamed-of goal. It beats counting calories!

● I want to change my life by _____ .
Insert short-term goal here (e.g., drinking less alcohol).

● In five years, as a result of my efforts, I would love to _____
_____ .
Insert long-term goals here (e.g., rely less on downing Cosmopolitans to have a good time).

● To get myself ready, I need to _____ ,
_____ and _____ .
Insert three things you can do right now to get closer to your goal (e.g., devote more time to
non-alcohol-related activities, like going to the theater).

● Knowing me, _____ ,
_____ and _____
Be brutally honest about three possible pitfalls here.
will get in my way, so I have to be prepared to _____ ,
_____ and _____ .
List three ways you'll avoid said pitfalls.

● To truly change, I need to make different choices every day, such as
being sure to _____ , _____
_____ and _____ .
List three doable strategies for sticking to your goal.

● Fortunately, I plan to reward myself by _____ ,
_____ and _____ .
Whatever revs your engine!

🕐 GOT 15 MINUTES?
Map things out

PUT YOUR DREAMS within your grasp with this exercise, based on a technique developed by Tony Buzan, author of *Age-Proof Your Brain* (Harper Thorsons). To begin, you'll need paper and colored markers.

1 Imagine an idyllic experience from your past (say, a moonlit stroll on the beach on your last vacation). This is the feeling you're seeking; keep it in mind.

2 Write *My perfect life* in a circle in the center of the page, then note all the things that includes (*buy house, write novel, have kids*), extending from the center like rays of the sun.

3 From each ray, draw branches labeled with your feelings and thoughts about that primary goal (for *write novel*, for example, you might jot down *teaching job* and *screenplay*). From each of those phrases, draw another line and do the same (from *teaching job,* for example, you might write *rewarding*; from *screenplay,* you might write *money*).

4 Highlight similar ideas in the same color; the dominant hues are goals you should aim for. If it's clear you yearn for creativity in your life, you might decide to take a painting class or join a museum.

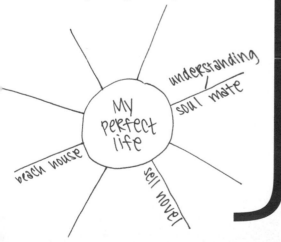

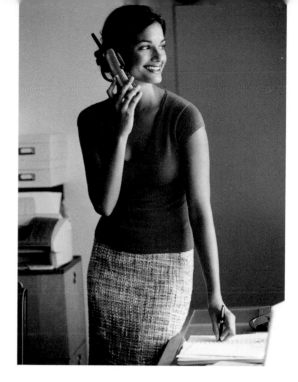

🕐 GOT 4 MINUTES?
Feel more connected

We all have days when we want to crawl right back into bed. Prep for them in advance by forming your own personal cheerleading squad: Identify three different people you can count on to improve your mood in a pinch. Program their numbers into speed dial. When you're feeling overwhelmed, glum or demoralized, work the phones. "Hearing pals' positive encouragement will lift your spirits," says Jan Yager, Ph.D., a sociologist in Stamford, Connecticut.

🕐 GOT 12 MINUTES?
Make a resolution that sticks—finally!

Instead of promising to stop doing something as you face a new year, fill your annual resolutions list with things you want to start doing: learn French, train for a mini-triathlon, travel to Malaysia. To make this the year your vows stick, use the following strategies:
KEEP THEM VISIBLE Stash resolutions on slips of paper in your desk, or tape them to your mirror.
SPREAD THE WORD Let your family know of your bold and brilliant plans so they can check in with you.
VISUALIZE YOUR SUCCESS See yourself making a toast to friends next New Year's Eve—in French!

🕐 GOT 10 MINUTES?
Improve the quality of your downtime

Don't waste another minute mindlessly surfing TV channels. You'll feel more satisfied if you use your free time doing relaxing things that engage you. Make a list of four quick-and-dirty ways you unwind that tend to leave you feeling fatigued or dissatisfied. Next, list some alternatives more likely to engage you. Or consider the following:

INSTEAD OF	TRY THIS
Watching reality TV	Document your reality with a blog, or send weekly e-mail updates with goofy or beautiful photos to far-flung friends.
Eating a bag of Oreos	Head to the kitchen to develop your own walnut brownie recipe or cook up your grandma's famous grasshopper pie.
Trolling the local mall	Host a "new to you" clothes-swapping party, where you and pals exchange garments that you no longer wear, or simply deconstruct some old T-shirts. You'll not only end up with a new outfit, but you'll save wear and tear on your credit card.
Playing a video game	Organize a rousing poker night with a group of your closest girlfriends. You can serve those special brownies you've developed, show off your new-old clothes and catch up on all the gossip. It's a nice change from dinner at a local restaurant.

🕐 GOT 10 MINUTES? Define your core values

It's easy to forget what truly matters in life. Remind yourself with this exercise from Dan Baker, Ph.D., founding director of the Life Enhancement Program at Canyon Ranch spa in Tucson, Arizona.

1 Circle the five qualities you value most.

Adventurousness	Empathy	Kindness
Artistry	Faithfulness	Love
Boldness	Fitness	Loyalty
Charity	Flexibility	Perceptiveness
Cheerfulness	Health	Pleasure
Civility	Helpfulness	Reverence
Cleanliness	Honesty	Simplicity
Compassion	Humility	Thrift
Courage	Humor	Trustworthiness
Creativity	Intelligence	Wealth
Dependability	Inventiveness	Wisdom

2 For each trait you circle, write a sentence describing how you usually incorporate it into each day: "I'm on time" for dependability, say.

3 Rank each from 1 to 5 based on how well you live by it (1 is not at all; 5, very much so).

4 Write small ways you can practice your lowest-ranked value (i.e., if adventurousness is last, you might write "Try a different cuisine this week" or "Plan a trip somewhere exotic").

YOUR HAPPINESS TO-DON'T LIST

» **Don't obsess** over your bank account. Studies suggest that people who do tend to be less happy.

» **Don't wait** for someone else to remember your birthday. Plan an outing with a friend and go enjoy!

» **Don't spill** all your secrets. No one has to know that you get a charge from rearranging your linen closet.

» **Don't stifle** a chuckle. As the saying goes, laughter *is* the best medicine.

» **Don't feel guilty** about taking a personal day. Use it to lie around the house or go shopping—for yourself!

» **Don't reply** to every e-mail note. Answer crucial ones; ignore the rest.

» **Don't spare compliments.** Let loved ones know you appreciate them and watch them light up. You will, too.

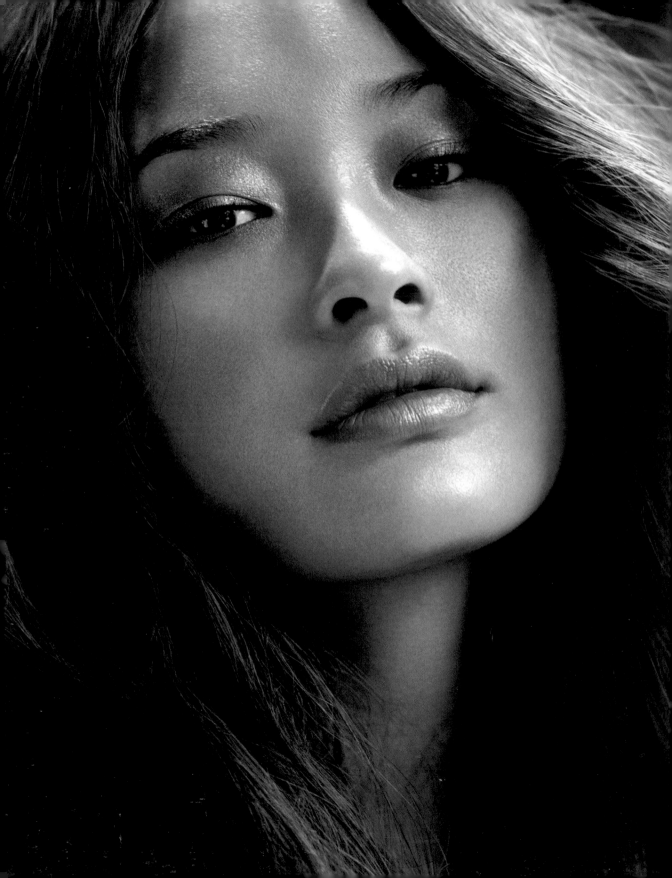

beauty boosters

CHAPTER
5

Healthy eating and fitness habits help you feel good from the inside out, but beauty works in the other direction. Nothing gives you unshakable confidence like skin so clear you don't need concealer. The best part: Looking and feeling terrific doesn't require an entire morning's investment. You can get hair that gleams, eyes that sparkle and skin that shouts "I'm healthy!" in minutes with this head-to-toe guide.

The only 10 things you need to know to look dazzlingly glowing and gorgeous

Want another incentive to take care of yourself? The basics of beauty start with a healthy lifestyle. Live by these principles and you'll achieve radiant skin, shiny hair and all the other hallmarks of looking good. The rest—a little lip gloss, a fun hairstyle—is icing on the cake.

1 Eat right

We'll cut straight to it: If you're eating nothing but junk and drinking everything but water, your skin will eventually show it by turning dull and dry or by breaking out. You can find nutrition strategies in chapter 3, but here's the main dish: Eat fruit and veggies; they're the chief source of antiaging antioxidants such as beta-carotene. Take in essential fatty acids, which help keep skin resilient. Get calcium so your teeth stay strong. And eat whole grains instead of white bread and white rice. When you digest refined carbs, your body pumps out extra insulin. It's not known why, but this hormone causes skin to retain fluids, possibly leading to blotches, puffiness and irritation.

2 Let go of stress

Stress not only frazzles nerves, but it also does a number on your looks. When you're feeling tense, your body releases cortisol, which may increase oil production in both skin and hair, making you susceptible to pimples and a greasy scalp. (In some people, it triggers the opposite reaction, sapping skin and hair of moisture.) Your nails may also grow more slowly and weaken. So take a yoga class, go for a stroll, focus on deepening your breathing, get a laugh—anything that pushes your personal PAUSE button. It will do your body good in more ways than one.

3 Catch 40 winks

It's not called beauty sleep for nothing. Aim for seven to nine hours a night. That's when skin repairs itself. A study in *The Journal of Investigative Dermatology* found that lack of rest can decrease skin's rate of renewal, giving it a dull look. Besides, rest helps you feel good, and that always makes you look better.

4 Use protection

The secret to smooth skin isn't a $90-a-drop magic serum. It's (drumroll, please) sunscreen! Slather it on every day to prevent premature wrinkles, not to mention skin cancer. No matter how good you think a tan looks, the long-term results—enlarged pores, brown spots, rough skin—won't be so attractive.

5 Make a clean sweep

To truly glow, you must be sparkly clean. Wash your face for a full 30 to 60 seconds to give cleansing agents time to loosen dirt, oil and makeup. Use a cleanser with scrubbing beads—or a bit of elbow grease. "People imitate TV ads, where models barely touch their faces, but you need a little friction," says Jeffrey Dover, M.D., associate clinical professor of dermatology at Yale University in New Haven, Connecticut. And be sure to rinse well. Residue can cause dry skin.

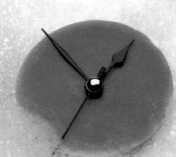

6 Exfoliate, exfoliate, exfoliate

Working out isn't the only secret to a bare-able body. You've got to have smooth, sexy skin. The road to radiance starts by sloughing off excess dead skin cells. (These cells dull the skin's surface because they don't reflect light.) Rely on body scrubs, or lather up with a hydrating body wash and exfoliate with a loofah. Using light pressure is key. Overscrubbing removes oils, and skin may become oilier to compensate. On dry spots, also go easy; harsh sloughing may irritate skin and it will thicken to protect itself. After you wash, rub in a lotion with salicylic acid. The acid continues to gently exfoliate, helping skin look even-toned.

7 Take care of your hair

Healthy hair is gorgeous hair, whether it's straight or curly, long or short, light or dark. Shine strategies that work: Get a trim every six to eight weeks so ends are less damage prone. Wash hair every other day so it can retain its natural oils, which help prevent frizz and flyaways. And apply a conditioner from the middle of hair shafts to the ends; oil glands at your scalp will moisturize the hair near your roots. Finally, wear your hair in a way that fits your lifestyle and personality. Don't ask for a cut that takes an hour to style if you're a wash-and-go kind of gal.

8 Accentuate your best feature

Natural beauty doesn't require that you swear off makeup. Simply follow the less-is-more principle. Instead of highlighting every gorgeous feature (which is overwhelming), choose your single best one to play up. To emphasize glowing skin, press a fingerprint of cream blush on cheeks and rub. To define lovely eyes, blend a deep-hued shadow along your top lash line. Curl lashes and apply mascara. For dramatic lips, fill them in with a creamy pencil and add a splash of color.

9 Find the right fragrance

Like makeup, perfume lets you express yourself without saying a word. In addition to sending a message to others (sexy or sweet?), it affects your mood. Research reveals that aromas can conjure positive memories. And certain scents have mood-changing power. Peppermint can distract you from

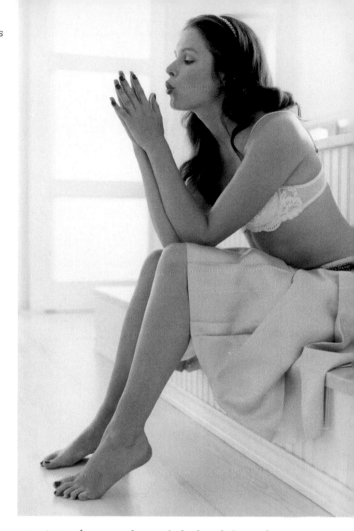

pain. Lavender can make you feel relaxed. (It produces beta waves in the brain, which is the first step in falling asleep.) Choose a scent, spritz one wrist, then touch wrists together. (Rubbing can alter the fragrance.)

10 Mind your hands and feet

By no means must you have a perfect mani and pedi 24/7. But healthy and hydrated digits do make a difference. Peeling, dry cuticles turn even the nicest nails ragged. And trimming (or, OK, biting) causes hangnails that look lousy and—ouch!—hurt like crazy. So apply cream often. One that contains dimethicone locks in moisture but isn't greasy. Brush nails in the shower to sweep away dirt, then gently push back cuticles. Get rid of excess dead skin by rubbing in a cuticle-remover gel. Rinse, then massage in oil. If you have time, apply nail-strengthening polish (even clear will do) to help prevent brittleness. You're good to go!

GOT 2 MINUTES?
Glow naturally
Coat fingers with lotion, then try this radiance-infusing massage.

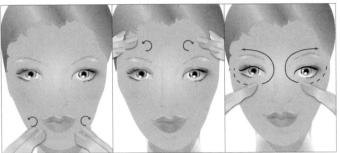

1 From your chin's center, make small circular motions along your jawline, then from above your lips to ears, and from the sides of your nose along your cheekbones.

2 Move your fingers to the middle of your forehead and massage again, moving slowly outward to your temples. Return to center, then repeat the process twice.

3 From your temples, glide along your eye socket bones, moving under your eyes, up the bridge of your nose, over your brows and back to your temples.

GOT 1 MINUTE?
Wash your face in a flash

Hate the extra step of using a separate makeup remover? Wash with a textured, foaming cleansing cloth instead. Or use a damp washcloth with your regular cleanser. The light friction removes your makeup better than cleanser alone and will leave your skin bright and healthy.

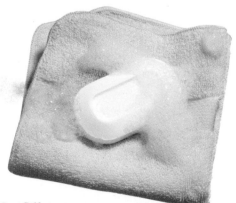

GOT 2 MINUTES?
Determine how old your skin really is
Take this quiz to assess the damage you've accrued and what you've been able to avoid.

Begin with your age ____

Do you have any brown spots or broken blood vessels? If yes, +2 ____

Are there noticeable lines around your eyes or lips? If yes, +3 ____

Do you see deep creases on your forehead or cheeks? If yes, +5 ____

Did you or do you tan—indoors or out—at least twice a week? If yes, with sunscreen, +5; if yes, without, +10 ____

Has your face suffered at least three peeling sunburns? If yes, +5 ____

Do you smoke? If yes, +3 ____

Do you drink five or more alcoholic beverages a week? If yes, +2 ____

If you answered no to every question, congrats! Your skin is the same age as you. If you said yes to any, move on.

Focus on prevention. **Start with the age you just determined and subtract the following:**

Do you work out at least three times a week? If yes, −1 ____

Do you munch on fruit and veggies three times each day? If yes, −1 ____

Do you use a product with SPF 15 each morning? If yes, −4 ____

Do you use antiaging creams (retinol or vitamin C)? If yes, −1 ____

Do you use prescription lotions (such as Retin-A)? If yes, −3 ____

YOUR SKIN'S AGE _____
To keep your complexion dewy, adopt the preventive behaviors above, and see the chart at right.

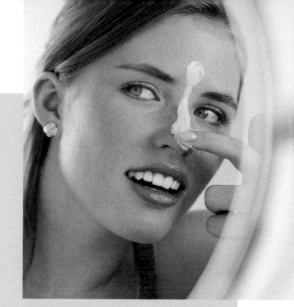

🕐 GOT 6 MINUTES?

Find a smooth-skin plan

Select your skin's main issue, then see how to resolve it. As the treatments get more powerful and effective, the potential for irritation increases, so follow the tips on how to help skin cope.

Your skin	What to use	How to use it	Insider tip
Slightly dull or rough; you want a fresh, brighter complexion.	An exfoliating peel pad or lotion with glycolic acid	Swipe skin with a peel pad for an instant glow. For longer-term results, apply a low-strength (5 percent) lotion once a day.	Mild tingling is OK; if skin stings, discontinue use. If skin isn't smoother in two weeks, return the lotion for a higher strength.
Rough texture and fine lines, or you want to prevent them.	A retinol night cream	Begin with a 0.03 percent or regular formula. Rub in a pea-sized drop every other night for the first two weeks, then every night.	Wait five minutes for the retinol to absorb, then apply lots of your usual moisturizer to prevent dryness and flakes.
Wrinkles or very uneven texture and tone, or you're over 30.	A prescription retinoic acid	See your derm for retinol's stronger sister. Follow the advice above in the retinol section to deal with initial peeling and redness.	Slather on a lotion with niacinamide (a form of vitamin B₃) before and during use of the Rx to help lessen side effects.

🕐 **GOT 1 MINUTE? Upgrade your moisturizer**

Review labels for these top hydrators. The more you see, the better.
- Glycerin and hyaluronic acid hold water molecules to skin's surface.
- Plant oils, dimethicone and petrolatum sit on skin and trap water.
- Ceramides and niacinamide strengthen skin's barrier so water stays in.

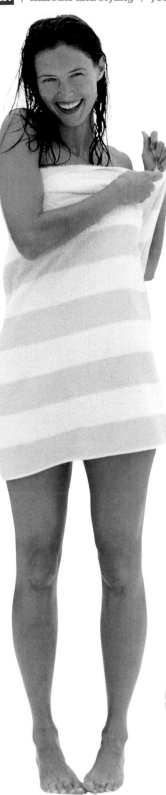

⏱ GOT 6 MINUTES?
Shampoo smarter

A lackadaisical wash may leave residue on your strands that can flatten your style. Try these easy tips for maximum shine and bounce.

1 Get soaked. More water means more lather, which distributes the shampoo through hair.

2 Use a shampoo that's free of sodium lauryl sulfate (check the label), which can strip hair of natural oils. Rub it between your palms and massage it in, starting at your nape. Then spend extra time around your temples and hairline, two often-oily areas that people tend to skip or speed over.

3 Concentrate on your roots, where hair is oiliest, but don't ignore the ends. The oldest, most porous part of your hair attracts the most dirt and product buildup. Pull up ends and massage with the rest of your hair. Lather for two to three minutes total.

4 Rinse completely by lifting hair at the roots and tousling until the water runs clear and free of suds. Hair may look dull if any shampoo is left behind.

5 Follow with conditioner. First, squeeze excess H_2O from hair because water-soaked strands can prevent absorption. Apply by walking conditioner-coated hands up from the ends.

6 Once you're out of the shower, lightly blot hair with a towel, but don't rub. Rubbing will roughen the strand's cuticle (its outer layer) and create frizz. Repeat these steps every other day, or daily if hair is oily or needs extra body.

⏱ GOT 2 MINUTES?
Scrub your scalp

Mix 1 tablespoon baking soda into 2 tablespoons shampoo and lather up. The soda exfoliates and absorbs oil for a superclean effect.

⏱ GOT 5 MINUTES?
Boost the volume of limp hair

If your style is too straight or deflates easily, make an appointment for highlights. Color roughens and swells strands for no-fuss texture.

⏱ GOT 1 MINUTE?
Strengthen hair while you get strong

Before working out, dampen hair, comb in conditioner, then put it in a ponytail or cover with a bandanna. Increased body heat from exercising will help hair absorb the product. Rinse post–sweat session.

GOT 30 SECONDS?
Examine your ends
If the ends of your hair are split or lighter in tone than the portion nearer your roots, it's time for a quarter-inch trim to prevent further breakage down the road.

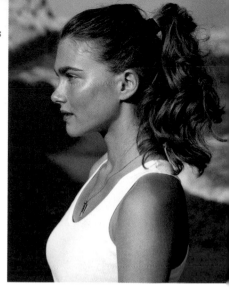

GOT 1 MINUTE?
Pick a perfect conditioner
Overwhelmed by all the bottles lining the hair aisle? Consult this chart to make shopping a breeze.

HAIR TYPE	HAIR FIX
Damaged	Protein-rich conditioners fill in cracks in the cuticle so it's stronger and smoother. A flat cuticle makes hair shiny because the smooth surface reflects more light.
Dry and frizzy	Oil and serum deep conditioners penetrate better than heavy masks. Apply one to dry hair (water and oil don't mix) before you go to bed, then rinse in the morning.
Limp or oily	Pick a volumizing conditioner and use on wet hair. Wait two minutes, rinse, then shampoo. The moisturizers penetrate, but you'll wash away hair-flattening heaviness.

GOT 12 MINUTES?
Style hair the healthy way

When you buy products, choose those that don't contain alcohol. Overdoing it on gel, mousse or other formulas with the ingredient can dry out hair.

Before you brush, lubricate towel-dried hair with a leave-in conditioner or detangler. Tearing through tangles can break vulnerable strands.

Prior to using heat from a dryer or flatiron, coat damp hair with a thermal leave-in spray, which protects from damage and adds shine.

While blow-drying, never rest the dryer's nozzle on your hair or on the brush bristles. Holding the nozzle 3 inches away will dry hair without scorching it.

If you wear a ponytail, switch the position of the elastic often—even if only a half inch up or down. "Hair can break in an elastic, causing flatness and flyaways in the area you always put it," says Cristophe, owner of five salons around the world.

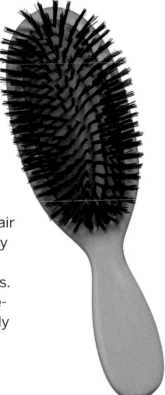

GOT 1 MINUTE?
Know your tools
Brushes and combs do more than detangle. If hair gets greasy, brush with boar bristles. They distribute oil down the hair shaft, giving you naturally lustrous, moisturized strands from roots to tips. In the shower, use a wide-tooth comb to help evenly distribute conditioner.

⏱ GOT 12 MINUTES?

Get a better blowout
Follow these steps to a sleek style.

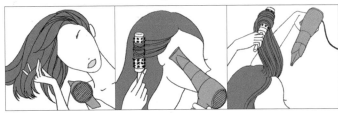

1 On damp hair, apply mousse or gel for hold, then cream to keep strands smooth. Dry 60 percent, fluffing with your fingers and lifting up at the roots.

2 Finish drying hair in six sections. For lift, pull them out or up from your scalp. Also, aim the dryer down hair shafts. It flattens the cuticle to add shine.

3 Hold the top sections up. Dry roots first, which trains hair to stand up rather than lie flat to your scalp. After hair is dry, spritz on hairspray.

⏱ GOT 7 MINUTES?

Create bouncy, frizz-free curls

APPLY THE RIGHT PRODUCTS In your palm, mix dime-sized drops of styling cream (to defrizz) and gel (for hold). Finger comb into damp hair from roots to tips.

SHAPE YOUR RINGLETS Once strands are coated, twirl small sections around a finger to give your curls shape. It's best to let curly hair air-dry, but if you're in a hurry, you can use a diffuser.

KEEP YOUR HANDS OFF Whatever drying method you choose, don't touch hair. Handling the curls can break them up and cause frizz—even after your hair is dry.

⏱ GOT 2 MINUTES? Assemble a happy-hair kit

Thirty percent of women say they have more bad-hair days than good. Head off an impending mane meltdown by keeping these 'do-good tools on hand.

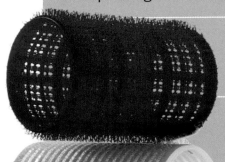

Cordless curling iron Pros defrizz with a round brush and blow-dryer. Do it with less effort (and one hand) with a curling iron that features a brush attachment.

No-snag elastics Fabric-wrapped elastics prevent breakage. For a quick fix, secure damp hair into a sleek, low ponytail or pull it halfway through for a chignon.

Velcro rollers Need to give your limp hair a lift? Heat dry strands with a blow-dryer for 30 seconds and set rollers close to the root. Leave them in for 10 minutes.

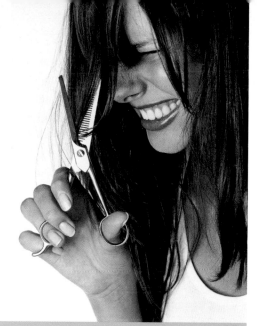

GOT 5 MINUTES?
Plan a hair makeover
Ready to go for something new? Whether you want a short style or long look, keep these tips in mind when talking to your stylist and together you'll come up with a flattering cut for you.

HAIR TYPE	IF YOU WANT A SHORT STYLE	IF YOU WANT TO KEEP HAIR LONG
STRAIGHT 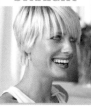	**Go for a pixie with long bangs** (at left). Fine or thin strands can seem lifeless when worn long. This spunky crop lets you ditch the deadweight but maintains some layers on top to prevent a Q-tip effect and keep the look modern.	**Love layers.** Layers frame your face, break up a curtain of long hair and help create texture, movement and volume. Keeping them many different lengths, not only two or three, looks even more appealing. Plus, light layers around your crown give lift to roots.
CURLY 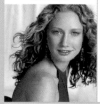	**Try a shoulder dusting bob.** Too-short curls may make you think Orphan Annie. And, unlike cropped cuts, a bob sustains its shape as hair grows. You'll also be able to tie hair back, but it's short enough that curls will stay bouncy, not weighed down.	**Lose the layers.** Traditional layers create a pyramid shape: flat on top and too full on the bottom. Instead, ask for a textured cut (at left)—hair that is sheared in long sections on an angle—so curls fit into each other like a puzzle, distributing the volume and bulk.
COARSE 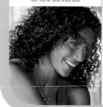	**Consider a pixie.** The cut can free you from relaxing treatments. Extra length on top—styled spiky, not sleek—makes a Mia Farrow hairstyle hip. Use creamy pomades or matte sprays to style; hair wet with wax or gel looks unfinished.	**Opt for a midlength look** (at left). Styling is more manageable when you have less bulk, so have your hairstylist remove some weight from the bottom and back with a razor. Don't let hair fall any longer than a few inches past your collarbone or the top may flatten.

GOT 7 MINUTES? Achieve loose, beachy waves
Separate dry hair into four sections and braid each (the more braids, the tighter the curls). Run a flatiron over each braid, then let them sit for a few minutes. Undo hair, tousle and apply shine spray to fight frizz.

🕐 GOT 13 MINUTES?

Be silky-smooth from head to toe Bikini season or not, these tips let you cultivate a beach-ready bod.

Thighs and butt

The quickest way to diminish the dimples of cellulite: Apply self-tanner. It evens out skin tone so bumps seem smoother. Glow lotions (moisturizers with a little DHA, the ingredient in self-tanner) let you gradually build color. The process is fast and virtually streakproof.

Back Prone to dreaded bacne? Traces of

conditioner may spur or exacerbate breakouts. Soap up after you condition, and after you shower, put on a robe or pin up hair to keep strands off your back. Treat breakouts with a benzoyl peroxide bar soap. After sudsing, wait a few seconds for skin to absorb the ingredient before you rinse.

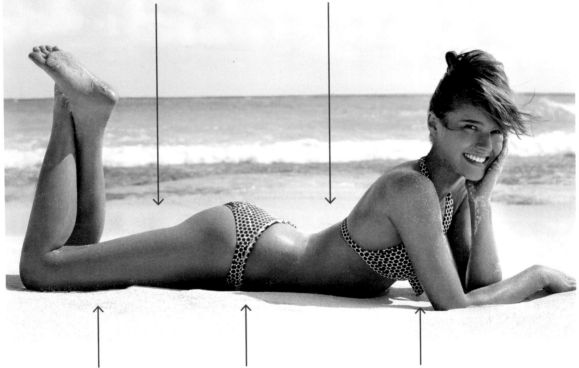

Legs If your legs get dry and

flaky, avoid soap and seek body washes with the same ingredients as those found in moisturizers: petrolatum, oils and shea butter. Also rub on a lotion or cream before you go to bed. At night, your body temperature rises, which helps skin soak up moisturizer.

Bikini line Prevent and

treat ingrown hairs following a wax or shave by swiping the area with a salicylic acid acne pad every other day. The beta hydroxy acid penetrates hair follicles to clear the debris that causes bumps. It also helps reduce inflammation if you already have them.

Arms Tiny, red bumps on the

back of arms are called keratosis pilaris. They occur when a buildup of dead skin cells form plugs that become inflamed and raised. Gently slough the area using a body wash with fine buffing beads. Follow with a moisturizer that contains exfoliating alpha or beta hydroxy acids.

GOT 30 SECONDS?
Ditch winter itch
Skin can get itchy when the temperature and humidity drop. Calm skin by mixing a 1 percent hydrocortisone cream 50-50 with your lotion.

⏱ GOT 6 MINUTES?
Remain sweat-free
Do you endure wetness despite using antiperspirant? Try these two tips:
● Apply your antiperspirant at night. The longer it stays in contact with your skin before you start perspiring, the better it will work.
● Towel-dry your pits after a bath or shower, then wait five minutes before you apply antiperspirant. The sweat-stopping ingredients won't absorb as well into waterlogged follicles.

⏱ GOT 2 MINUTES?
Keep cool
Lather up with body washes containing peppermint or camphor, a cooling herb (it's a main ingredient in Vicks VapoRub). Your skin will be refreshed even after you dry off.

⏱ GOT 7 MINUTES?
Exfoliate effortlessly
Don't wait 20 minutes for a body mask to work. Fill the bathtub, rub it on as the tub fills, and hop in. The mask smooths skin while you soak.

⏱ GOT 12 MINUTES?
Draw a mind-calming, skin-smoothing bath
Follow these four steps for a relaxing, spa-ahhh experience at home.

1 Trade the high-watt bulbs in your bathroom for candles. Research suggests that bright light may inhibit the production of melatonin, a hormone that helps induce sleep.

2 Fill your tub with warm, not hot, water. If it's scalding or you have to get used to the temperature, you may find it difficult to relax.

3 Add a couple of tablespoons of magnesium-rich Dead Sea salts. The minerals may help reduce inflammation and hydrate skin.

4 Pour in two capfuls of bath oil to add moisture. Or stand in the tub and massage in an oily salt scrub. Then, when you lie down and relax, the salt dissolves, but the oil will remain and keep skin supple.

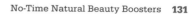

🕐 GOT 15 MINUTES?
Give yourself a spot check

Each month, scan for moles and bumps. Look on your scalp, between toes, everywhere. Print a copy of this body map at Self.com/go/tools to help you track new and changing ones. Use the pictures to learn what's suspect; if you find any that seem similar, see a derm.

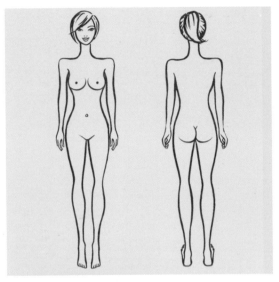

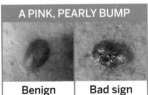

A PINK, PEARLY BUMP

| Benign | Bad sign |

Basal cell carcinoma is the most common type of skin cancer. It usually resembles a pearly bump or a sore that won't heal.

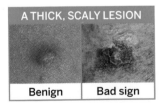

A THICK, SCALY LESION

| Benign | Bad sign |

Squamous cell carcinoma, the next most common, can be a red or flesh-toned bump that's raised and crusty.

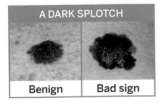

A DARK SPLOTCH

| Benign | Bad sign |

Melanoma can be fatal. Watch for an asymmetrical shape, irregular borders, uneven color and a large diameter.

🕐 GOT 1 MINUTE?
Rub on backup SPF

Even if your makeup contains sunscreen, you can't count on it for full protection. Many people spot-cover or only apply a light coat. And after two hours, foundation may shift, leaving uneven coverage. The effortless way to shield skin: Wear a moisturizer with an SPF of 15 or higher every day. If you don't like the feel of it under makeup, give your skin 10 minutes to absorb the lotion before applying foundation, and skin will feel less greasy.

🕐 GOT 4 MINUTES?
Wear enough sunscreen

The majority of people put on only about half the sunscreen needed to reach the labeled SPF of their lotion. If you have a hard time visualizing a 1-ounce dose, try this trick: Squeeze a thick line down each arm (use this to cover your chest, too) and each leg, then two lines down your back and stomach, and rub. If it seems goopy, go for two lighter layers one after the other.

GOT 30 SECONDS?

Understand UV rays
Ultraviolet A (UVA) rays are present all day and age skin. UVB rays (worst at midday) burn. Broad-spectrum sunscreen protects you from both.

⏱ GOT 3 MINUTES?

Become sun smart How to stay safe by the numbers

1 Ounces of sunscreen you need to cover your entire body. (Think of a shot glass.)

2 Hours between sunscreen applications if you're outside. Even a high SPF won't protect you all day.

3 Years a bottle of sunscreen lasts on the shelf, on average; lotions kept in a hot car or in the sun may not last as long.

6 Hours during the day (between 10 A.M. and 4 P.M.) when the sun's rays are strongest. Wear a hat and long sleeves, or stay in a shaded area if possible.

20 Percentage chance you'll be diagnosed with skin cancer in your lifetime. If you are Caucasian, your risk jumps to 33 percent.

30 Minutes before sun exposure you need to apply sunscreen for full protection. Skin needs time to absorb it, so don't wait until you get outside.

40 Minutes a water-resistant sunscreen protects while you're in the water. Waterproof lotion protects for 80 minutes. Reapply after toweling off.

80 Percentage you reduced your risk for skin cancer if you used sunscreen regularly as a kid. If you have children, slather or spray them often.

93 Percentage of rays a sunscreen with an SPF of 15 blocks. A lotion with SPF 30 blocks about 97 percent. Have a choice? Pick the latter; every bit counts.

100 Percentage chance that you need sunscreen if it's daytime. UV rays penetrate clouds and bounce off water, sand and other surfaces.

⏱ GOT 1 MINUTE? Help skin stay clear

Hate to wear sunscreen because you're convinced it makes you break out? Try a noncomedogenic, oil-free one made specifically for faces. Also, sunscreen can be tough to remove, especially waterproof formulas, so the pore-clogging residue may have been responsible for past breakouts. Solution: Wash with a cleansing scrub or a cloth with salicylic acid.

⏱ GOT 2 MINUTES?

Degrease your sunblock

To prevent an oil slick, in your hand, mix a bit of loose powder bronzer together with your facial sunscreen. It will help control shine and give you a golden, safe glow.

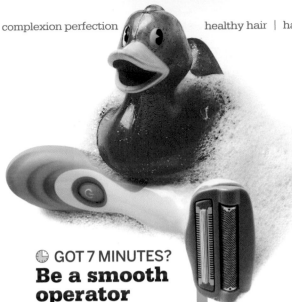

⏱ GOT 3 MINUTES?
Build a safe tan slowly

Glow lotions contain a small amount of DHA, the ingredient in self-tanner, making them a cinch to use. Just follow these success tips:

EXFOLIATE Even low levels of DHA can cause splotches where there are dry patches.

APPLY Smooth on lotion normally, and avoid vigorous rubbing. It can interfere with DHA.

PRESERVE Use a creamy body wash; it keeps skin hydrated and color from flaking.

⏱ GOT 7 MINUTES?
Be a smooth operator

Flaky skin and sunscreen can gum up your razor blade, so exfoliate before shaving. Prone to bumps? Shave down, in the direction hair grows.

⏱ GOT 10 MINUTES?
Stay silky

If you hate having to shave frequently, pick up one of these.

A depilatory melts hair right below skin's surface, keeping you smooth twice as long as shaving does. Try a no-drip gel with a bladeless razor, which squeegees off every last hair.

An at-home wax removes hair from the root, helping results last up to a month. Roll-ons and precoated strips are fast, easy and mess-free options.

⏱ GOT 1 MINUTE?
Wait to wax

Schedule your monthly wax appointment so it falls after your period. Things hurt less when estrogen levels are high.

⏱ GOT 15 MINUTES?
Wax your bikini line

Do-it-yourself upkeep saves time and money (plus an awkward encounter, if you're shy). It's not as painful as you think—really.

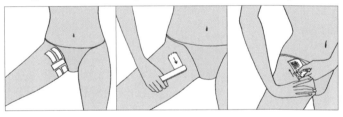

1 Prep skin by exfoliating the area with a scrub or washcloth and trimming hairs to a half inch. Then dust on powder, which prevents wax from sticking to skin. Mentally plan the sections you'll wax (and the order). Doing so makes the task easier to manage.

2 Opt for a wax roll-on, precoated strips or a kit that includes the wax, spatula, muslin strips and postwax oil. Apply wax to the first section in a layer thinner than a penny. Use the spatula's edge, as if buttering toast; the flat side goops on too much.

3 Rub on the muslin (or wax strip), leaving a pull tab. Hold skin taut with one hand and quickly pull back the cloth with the other. Keep it close to skin. Don't yank the strip up, which can hurt and break hairs. Press fingers to the area. Don't forget to breathe!

◍ GOT 15 MINUTES? Get a fabulous faux-glow from head to toe

Exfoliate with a loofah in the shower, then, before you reach for the self-tanner, check out these tricks to help bypass blotches and achieve a pro-quality bronzing.

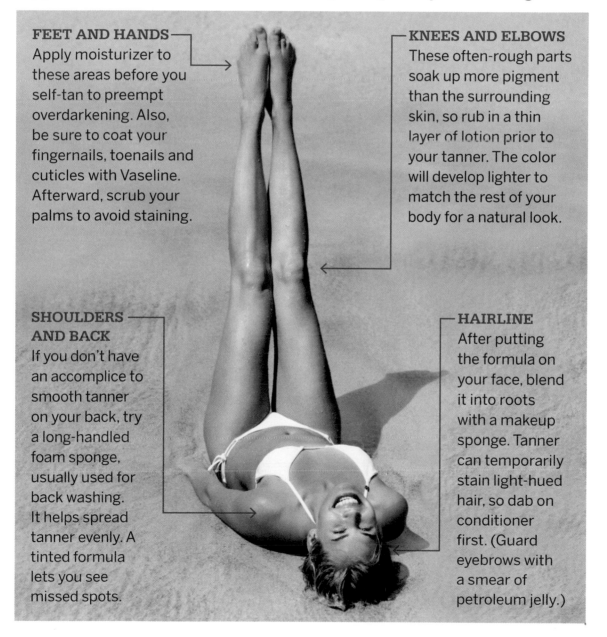

FEET AND HANDS Apply moisturizer to these areas before you self-tan to preempt overdarkening. Also, be sure to coat your fingernails, toenails and cuticles with Vaseline. Afterward, scrub your palms to avoid staining.

KNEES AND ELBOWS These often-rough parts soak up more pigment than the surrounding skin, so rub in a thin layer of lotion prior to your tanner. The color will develop lighter to match the rest of your body for a natural look.

SHOULDERS AND BACK If you don't have an accomplice to smooth tanner on your back, try a long-handled foam sponge, usually used for back washing. It helps spread tanner evenly. A tinted formula lets you see missed spots.

HAIRLINE After putting the formula on your face, blend it into roots with a makeup sponge. Tanner can temporarily stain light-hued hair, so dab on conditioner first. (Guard eyebrows with a smear of petroleum jelly.)

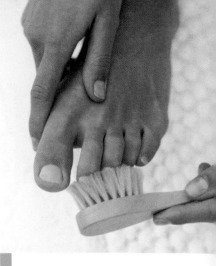

⏱ GOT 15 MINUTES?
Give yourself an at-home manicure or pedicure
Don't wait for an appointment! Get great nails on your own.

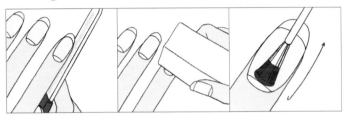

1 Clip overly long nails; filing straight across to shorten can leave them weakened. (And wait to wash hands or apply lotion; moisture separates your nails' layers, increasing the risk for splits and breaks.) Next, file the sides straight. Place the tool parallel to your finger. File the tips' corners using a rounded motion. As for nail shape, the curve should be a mirror image of your cuticle.

2 Put lotion inside two plastic sandwich bags and microwave them for three seconds. Insert your hands and relax for a few minutes. Toss the bags, rub in the excess lotion, then carefully push back your cuticles with a soft towel. Put down the nippers! Instead, apply oil and use a buffer to gently exfoliate your cuticles and nails. You slough off dead skin and keep the protective part intact.

3 Clean the surface of your nails with polish remover and brush on a base coat. It acts like double-sided tape, helping polish stick. Then, when applying color, splay out the brush above your cuticle (as shown). Move it down to the cuticle and out to the tip; this prevents the polish from welling up on skin. Repeat on either side for three swipes total. Paint all nails, add a second coat, then a top coat. Let dry.

⏱ GOT 10 MINUTES?
Smooth rough skin

Hands Rub an exfoliating face mask all over hands. They can tolerate a strong glycolic acid product, but if they're red and dry, go acid-free. Next, "wash" hands with a coarse scrub, spending extra time around cuticles, then put on lotion. Or turn chores into treatment time: Apply a mask of lotion and slip on rubber gloves before you get busy.

Feet Toss a fizzy bath bomb in a basin of water, add five drops of cuticle remover (to soften thick skin) and soak. Scrub feet with a grainy exfoliant. Use your thumb and the grains to scrub nail beds, too; this buffs them, adding a sheen. Rinse, then massage in cream.

⏱ GOT 3 MINUTES? Wear dark polish confidently
Deep red, plum and purple are chic shades, but they can also be intimidating. Keep the effect dramatic, not Dragon Lady, by filing nails short. Look at your palm: Nail tips should peek out just past fingers.

⏱ GOT 1 MINUTE?
Repair a smudge

One nicked tip or toe need not mean a ruined manicure. Maintain a perfect 10 with this handy advice.

SOAK IT Dip a cotton swab into polish remover. Dab it onto the pad of the index finger opposite the hand with the mussed manicure.

SWIPE IT Sweep the damp finger across the nicked nail several times. You'll thin and redistribute the polish, so there's no need to repaint.

SEAL IT Wait a few seconds until the nail is dry, then apply a clear top coat to lock in color and add shine.

⏱ GOT 1 MINUTE?
Pick nailcolor that lasts

Opt for shimmery formulas; they have bits of mica or crushed pearl, which anchor color to your nails.

⏱ GOT 2 MINUTES?
Choose a pretty color combo

Go bold on toes, but use a lighter hue in the same color family for your fingernails.

COLOR	TOES	FINGERS
If you opt for orange		
If you prefer pink		
If you're a purple person		

⏱ GOT 3 MINUTES?
Fight flakes Make a few simple changes to your routine to turn parched hands and feet pretty.

TRADE IN	TRY INSTEAD
Antibacterial hand washes Ingredients that fight bacteria, such as triclosan, can be drying.	**Creamy cleansers** Read the ingredients list for skin-conditioning additives such as glycerin.
Callus shavers and foot files Both tools can cause cuts that may lead to an infection.	**Exfoliating scrubs** Sugar scrubs have fine granules (gentler on hands). Save coarse salt or pumice for feet.
Light lotions Products with a whipped-cream consistency might not be enough on very dry skin.	**Heavy creams** Try for a texture like pudding or butter. One with petrolatum traps moisture to soften all day.

⏱ GOT 3 MINUTES?
Help your lipcolor last

Try one or all of these tips for a stay-put shade.

1 **Blend your foundation** over your lip line and lips so short-lived gloss and sheer lipsticks have something to grab on to.

2 **Fill in lips** with a neutral-colored pencil. (A soft, round-tip one won't feel dry.) Hold the pencil flat and shade with it rather than draw, then smudge the color with your finger to avoid a drawn-on effect.

3 **Blot lips** before applying lipstick or gloss because color adheres better to a moisture-free mouth. After swiping on one coat, blot again. You will remove the oils but leave pigment. Finish with a second coat.

4 **After applying lipstick,** hold a single sheet of Kleenex over your lips and brush on translucent powder. A fine dust will sift through and set the makeup.

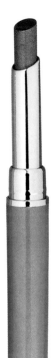

⏱ GOT 2 MINUTES?
Shine with shimmer

Sparkle is like chocolate; it's easy to overindulge. Stay subtle with these tricks.

● **Brighten eyes.** Brush shimmer shadow on your lash line only, and blend it up onto your lid with a finger dipped in Vaseline.

● **Raise cheekbones.** Lightly dot cream shimmer in a crescent shape from your temples to under the outer half of eyes.

⏱ GOT 1 MINUTE?
Blush flawlessly

PREP Dust translucent powder over liquid foundation. Powder blush adheres to moist skin and prevents even blending.

COLOR Pick a pink or more golden pinky-peach with a soft pearl effect. Apply to apples in an outward, circular motion.

⏱ GOT 5 MINUTES? Have a bright eye-dea

There are more types of makeup for eyes than for any other feature. Apply it gorgeously!

MAKEUP	MUST-KNOW HOW-TOS
Concealer	With a pointed brush, dab concealer on dark areas at the inner and outer corners of eyes. Gently blend with your finger; body heat helps cover-up melt into skin so it doesn't look cakey. Using a puff, press powder over the concealer to set.
Eyeliner	Nothing helps peepers pop like eyeliner. Choose a soft, creamy pencil, which goes on smoothly. Hold your lid taut and use short, feathering strokes, placing the pencil's tip between lashes for each new stroke. Then smudge with a brush.
Eyeshadow	Neutralize ruddy lids first by dabbing on yellow-toned eye primer or concealer. Apply shadow more intensely near your lash line and blend so it's lightest at the crease. This gradation approach looks more natural than a uniform wash of color.
Mascara	Curl lashes first. (Position the curler and pump for 10 seconds.) Remove globs from your mascara brush with a tissue. Comb mascara through lashes, turning the wand so all 360 degrees make a pass to fully coat and separate hairs.

🕐 GOT 2 MINUTES?

Find a foundation

The right base can take your skin from faulty to flawless. If you're not certain which formula is best, use this foolproof chart to make your complexion's dream match.

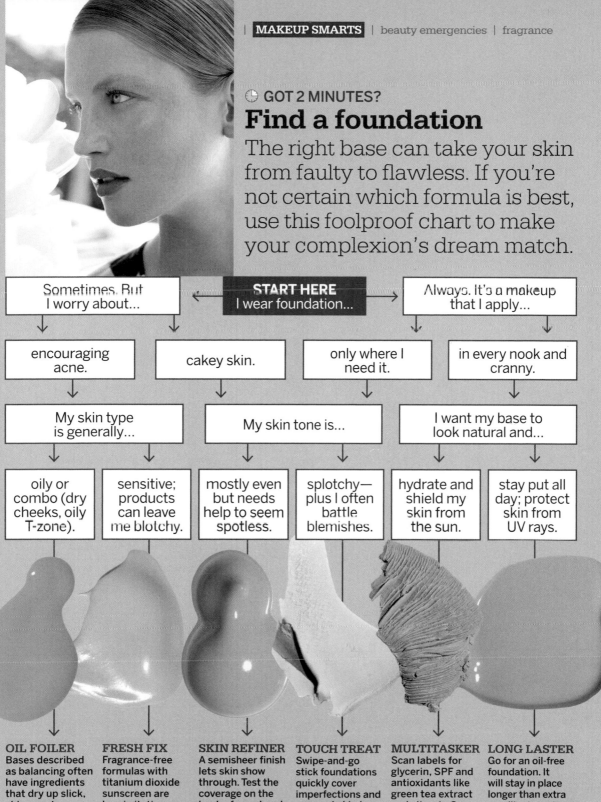

| Sometimes. But I worry about... | **START HERE** I wear foundation... | Always. It's a makeup that I apply... |

encouraging acne.

cakey skin.

only where I need it.

in every nook and cranny.

My skin type is generally...

My skin tone is...

I want my base to look natural and...

oily or combo (dry cheeks, oily T-zone).

sensitive; products can leave me blotchy.

mostly even but needs help to seem spotless.

splotchy— plus I often battle blemishes.

hydrate and shield my skin from the sun.

stay put all day; protect skin from UV rays.

OIL FOILER
Bases described as balancing often have ingredients that dry up slick, shiny spots.

FRESH FIX
Fragrance-free formulas with titanium dioxide sunscreen are less irritating.

SKIN REFINER
A semisheer finish lets skin show through. Test the coverage on the back of your hand.

TOUCH TREAT
Swipe-and-go stick foundations quickly cover imperfections and even out skin tone.

MULTITASKER
Scan labels for glycerin, SPF and antioxidants like green tea extract and vitamin C.

LONG LASTER
Go for an oil-free foundation. It will stay in place longer than extra emollient versions.

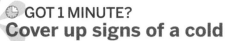

🕐 GOT 1 MINUTE?
Fix a blush blunder

Ever look in the mirror after applying cheek color only to realize you look more Bozo than beautiful? To lighten a heavy-handed application, dot concealer on top and blend. You'll soften the color without removing any foundation or sunscreen underneath.

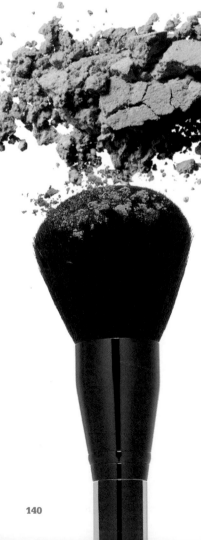

🕐 GOT 1 MINUTE?
Cover up signs of a cold

● Start with a tinted moisturizer, then top with foundation. A stick formulation has the most opacity to hide redness.
● Lock in coverage by dusting loose powder (ideally in the same shade as your base) over your nose.
● Your moisturizer's effects are likely to wear off in a few hours. To head off dryness, massage a drop of lotion onto your fingertips and press the thin layer on flaky areas.

🕐 GOT 4 MINUTES?
Care for a cut, prevent a scar

OLD FIX	NEW FIX
Hydrogen peroxide	Wash with soap and water. Cleaning your cut with peroxide slows healing because it stops the formation of new cells.
Air it out	Swab on petroleum jelly. Keeping the area moist will encourage cells to grow over the wound more quickly.
Adhesive bandage	Use an Adaptic bandage. A liquid bandage also works. The former keeps the pad from sticking to your scrape. The latter seals a cut.

🕐 GOT 2 MINUTES?
Look lovely after a long day

Need a rapid beauty-resuscitation plan? Read on.

1 Apply lotion to dry patches, blot shiny spots with tissue and wipe mascara from under your eyes.

2 Touch up or add more foundation or concealer around your nose and eyes and any blemishes.

3 Add extra blush for evening. Smooth eyeshadow creases, then apply eyeliner to your top lash line.

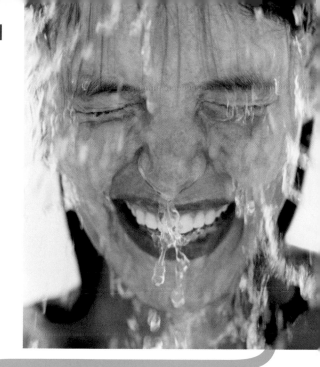

🕐 GOT 5 MINUTES?

Test your acne IQ

There are a lot of myths about what causes pimples. Learn the truth and stay in the clear.

1. Eating chocolate can make your skin break out.
☐ True ☐ False

2. Having frequent clusters of zits means skin is dirty.
☐ True ☐ False

3. Hair products could be to blame for skin problems.
☐ True ☐ False

4. To treat acne, you must dry up any oil on your face.
☐ True ☐ False

5. A salon facial will help rid you of pimples.
☐ True ☐ False

6. Getting some sun can clear up your skin.
☐ True ☐ False

Answers

1 FALSE But there is a connection between milk and acne, so avoid overdoing it on dairy.

2 FALSE If you hit the sack without cleansing, makeup, dirt and oil can clog pores, but persistent acne often comes from an abundance of bacteria. Wash with a cleanser that contains antibacterial triclosan.

3 TRUE Emollients in some styling products can rub off and plug pores. Try silicon-based products instead.

4 FALSE Dry skin isn't the answer, especially as you get older. Better: noncomedogenic products.

5 FALSE Steam used during a facial can swell skin's top layer, trapping oil and bacteria. Get a massage!

6 TRUE AND FALSE A little sun exposure may help, but heat can swell skin (like steam), trapping blemish breeders, not to mention the other harmful effects of UV.

🕐 **GOT 8 MINUTES?** Treat your type of breakout

Most women with breakouts fall into two categories. Find yours, then check out the right regimen.

PIMPLE PROFILE You get occasional zits, one to three at a time, that seem to take over your face.

- To keep pores clear, use a salicylic acid wash or pad every day or when you typically break out.
- If you have a red, swollen zit, look for a spot treatment with salicylic acid and sulfur, an anti-inflammatory that shrinks and calms pimples.
- On a whitehead, dab on salicylic acid gel, then a benzoyl peroxide spot treatment, which helps fight bacteria. You can wear the combo under makeup.

PIMPLE PROFILE No matter what, you always have bunches of red blemishes or whiteheads.

- Twice a day, cleanse with an over-the-counter triclosan (an antibacterial) and salicylic acid wash. Spend about 30 seconds sudsing, but don't scrub.
- Rub in a 2.5 percent benzoyl peroxide (BP) lotion (also OTC). A higher strength is more drying and may not work better. A sulfur mask can calm red spots.
- When acne subsides, continue with the wash and lotion. Wean yourself off the BP if it dries skin.

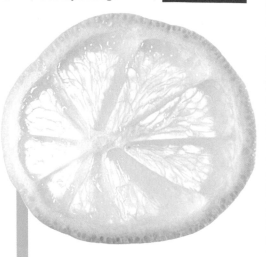

🕐 GOT 15 MINUTES?
Shop for perfume
In the market for a scent? Follow these tips so you will be more likely to come home with a new favorite.

1 Your sensitivity to scent increases throughout the day, so head to the store in the afternoon or evening.

2 Avoid wearing a perfumed lotion or spritzing near a watchband. Both can interfere with a fragrance.

3 Always sniff fragrance on a strip or something else before putting it on your skin. If you don't like it on paper, chances are it won't improve on you.

4 Wait to inhale. Most perfumes contain alcohol, which can temporarily dull your nose if you take a deep whiff right away. Spray a strip, wait 30 seconds for the alcohol to dissipate, then take a few short sniffs.

5 Don't test more than five perfumes in one session or you could overload—and confuse—your scent receptors. It's worth it to make a few shopping trips.

6 Everyone's body chemistry is different—you may love your mom's fragrance but find it doesn't work for you—so sample even familiar scents on your skin.

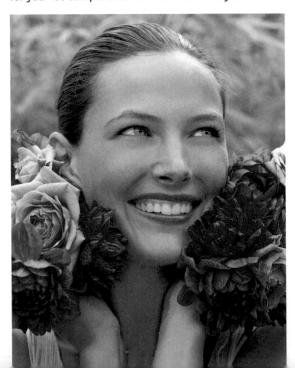

🕐 GOT 3 MINUTES?
Lighten a scent application
If you oversprayed, wash the area with soap and water, then grab a lemon. The acidic juice cuts the fragrance's oil. Soak a cotton ball in the juice and rub it over the area. Wash again, then spritz for a fresh start—and scent.

🕐 GOT 1 MINUTE?
Preserve your perfume
Stop! Don't toss that box. Keep the bottles you don't spritz often in their container and store in a cool, dark place. It helps the aroma stay true.

🕐 GOT 1 MINUTE?
Keep your scent work-appropriate
For perfume that is too strong for the office, spray it on a brush and run it through your hair. You'll soften and disperse the aroma, making it coworker-friendly.

YOUR BEAUTY TO-DON'T LIST

» **Don't shampoo** your hair every day. Overwashing zaps moisture and can make your strands frizzy and dry.

» **Don't buy** a magnifying mirror. Only a dermatologist needs to inspect your skin (and any flaws) that close up.

» **Don't overuse** teeth-whitening kits. Doing so can irritate gums and make teeth sensitive. Twice a year is plenty.

» **Don't soak** in long, hot showers or baths; it can dry out your skin.

» **Don't try to shape** your brows at home. Tweeze strays and hairs that fall in unibrow territory, but a pro will do a better job of full-on shaping.

» **Don't hit the tanning salon** for a protective base. There's no such thing. In fact, exposure to UV lamps is on the government's list of cancer causers.

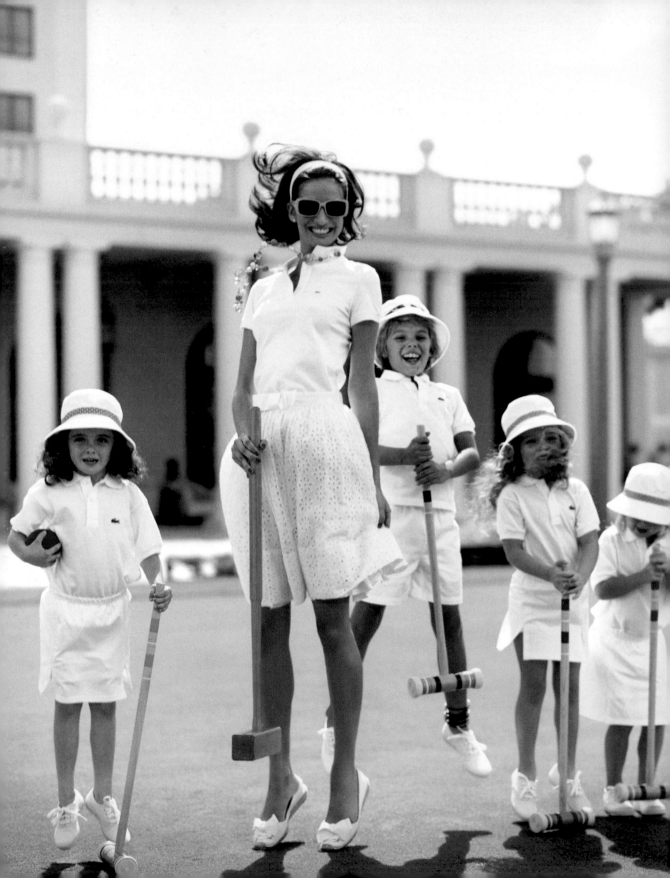

QUICKIE
style
secrets

You don't have to be a fashion editor or a big spender to dress comfortably, stylishly and with personal flair. The insider style tips on the next pages will teach you how to shop smarter, accessorize with ease, make off-the-rack clothes seem as if they're custom-tailored and get the most out of every dollar you spend on your wardrobe. You'll never stare blankly into your closet again.

The only 10 things you need to know to look stylish every time you leave the house

Nothing so instantly affects how other people see you and how you see yourself as what you wear. The clothing choices you make each morning help determine how your entire day will unfold: whether you'll feel confident and gorgeous or self-conscious and uncomfortable. With these simple rules, anyone—regardless of the shape of her body or the size of her budget—can look her best.

1 Own the go-to classics

Although they have their pick of clothes, most of SELF's fashion editors turn again and again to a few key pieces. Add these five classics to your closet and you can be well dressed in an instant.

● **A black sweater** It goes with everything. Buy crewneck or V-neck, whichever looks better on you. Splurge on cashmere of decent weight; your skin deserves it.

● **A crisp white shirt** One that buttons down the front (no button-down collar, no pockets) can be dressed up or down. Seriously, what else looks equally great over a bathing suit, with jeans and under a business suit?

● **A knee-length skirt** Select an A-line cut if you're pear-shaped or a straight, slim cut if you're top-heavy or hipless. Knee-length means it comes to the *top* of your knee, not the bottom. (That's the difference between looking sexy or schoolmarmish.)

● **A trench coat** Wear it on rainy days, sunny days, any day. It needn't be beige. A zingy color such as sunshine yellow turns a basic trench into a statement maker.

● **A simple handbag** Choose a solid color and a classic shape. A tan tote is more timeless than a striped, drawstring-topped duffle. Keep any clasps and buckles subdued so your bag will always be in style.

2 Shop with intention

If you shop willy-nilly, you risk ending up with lots of great clothes but not a single great outfit. (Ever bought the perfect top only to find you're missing the perfect pants to go with it?) Before you hit the mall, make a list of which items you're missing. Take along any pieces you're trying to match.

3 Don't obsess over size

First of all, being petite or plus-sized has nothing—zip! zilch! zero!—to do with how beautiful you are. Second of all, almost every designer these days uses a different sizing chart. You may be a 6 in one brand and a 10 in another. Buy what fits well and you'll feel gorgeous. Tear out the size tag.

4 Find a good tailor

Off-the-rack clothes are made to fit as many bodies as possible, which is good and bad. For example, designers know a 5-foot-2-inch woman and a 5-foot-9-inch woman might both buy their wrap dress in a size 8, but obviously, it won't fit them the same way. If you find an item you love, but it doesn't lie quite right, have it altered. Tailoring off-the-rack clothes to your body makes them seem like high-end pieces at a fraction of the cost.

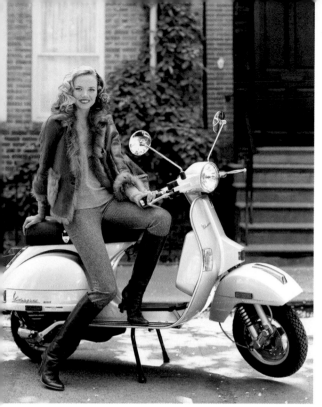

7 Follow trends judiciously

Not every new piece of clothing will flatter every body type. Know what works for you and stick with it. If the hot new must-have doesn't suit your shape, don't try to force it. The next trend is only a few sunsets away, and in the meantime, you can stay up-to-date by adding the latest accessories.

8 Mind your hem

Never wear the same pants with both heels and flats; your cuffs will either drag the ground or graze your ankles. Stock your closet with two lengths of trousers, so that whatever your heel height, your hem hangs a half inch off the floor.

9 Seek balance

Yes, make a fashion statement—just don't do it with every single part of your body.

• **Vary your proportions**. If you wear a woolly sweater on top, slip on tailored pants to avoid the Abominable Snowman effect. Conversely, if you put on a pleated or poufy skirt, pair it with a fitted top.

• **Accessorize in moderation.** If you wear elaborate earrings, opt for a simple chain necklace, or you risk looking like a Christmas tree. When you don a chunky choker, try small studs in your ears.

• **Mix textures.** Don't go head-to-toe tweed, denim, suede or anything. Unless you're wearing a suit, each piece of the outfit should look and feel different, yet complementary. If you feel as if you're camouflaged, swap out one or two of the items.

5 Splurge on your lingerie

Not only do quality underpinnings feel good on your skin and do wonders for your mood (you sexy thing!), but they also help your clothes hang better, giving you a smoother line. Some essentials:

• **A full slip in black or nude (or both)** To decide when to wear it, do a light check. Wearing the dress you've chosen, stand with a sunlit window behind you and a mirror in front. Is it see-through? Slip on the slip.

• **Seamless bras and undies** Panty lines and bra seams can ruin the look of clothes that fit you to a T.

• **Cute, colored camisoles** You'll stress less about your straps peeking out if they're pretty and lacy.

• **Black stockings** Go for high-quality, sheer ones. Shiny ones are for professional tap dancers only.

6 Listen to your baby toe

This information will be revolutionary for some of you, so read it very carefully: Never buy new shoes that don't feel comfortable when you try them on, thinking that when you get home you will break them in. It never works. Ever. Buy only shoes that fit well immediately and make your feet feel good, so the rest of you does, too.

10 Have fun

It's a simple principle, but it's so important. What you choose to wear is an expression of who you are and how you feel on that particular day. You can dress to feel powerful or demure, seductive or bashful, carefree or serious (even if on the inside you feel like none of those things!). Never be afraid to try something new. You might discover something exciting about yourself.

🕐 GOT 2 MINUTES?

Spot quality when you clothes shop

ASSESS ITEMS ON THE RACK Before you buy, "turn everything inside out," says stylist Star Klem of Nashville, who has worked with stars such as Ashley Judd. "A crooked seam creates a poor fit. If it looks as if I could have sewn it with my feet, I don't buy it."

SCAN FOR SHODDY STITCHING It's a telltale sign of cheaply made clothing. Don't be afraid to (gently!) pull at the seams to test their sturdiness. Be especially wary of stretchy fabrics. A stretch top made with non-stretch thread could fall apart easily or develop holes.

TRUST YOUR SENSE OF TOUCH When you see a garment you like on the rack, pay attention to the texture of the fabric. If it doesn't feel good on your fingers, then it won't feel good on your body.

NOTE THE COLOR Bright clothes and accessories can more easily look cheap than softer shades. "When you see knockoffs in the store, the colors are usually a lot punchier" than on the originals, explains Nicole Chavez, who often styles Rachel Bilson and Ashlee Simpson. "Muted colors translate to higher quality."

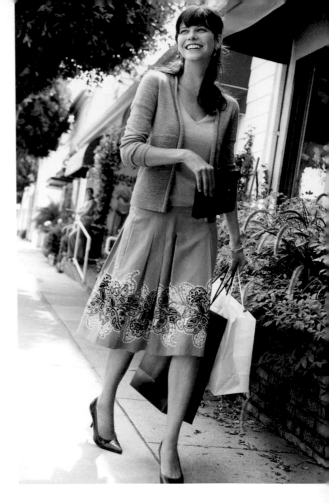

🕐 GOT 5 MINUTES?

Triple-check your decision

Don't head to the cashier with your style find until you've used this checklist to make sure you'll be happy with your purchase.

☐ **READ THE CARE LABEL** Are you prepared to hand wash, dry-clean or do whatever the instructions demand? If maintaining the item will be a burden, rethink your decision.

☐ **MOVE AROUND IN THE CLOTHES** If it's a pair of pants or a skirt, sit down and cross your legs or mime going up stairs. With a new shirt, move your arms around and swing your purse over your shoulder. An item that looks amazing as you pose in the dressing-room mirror might gap or feel uncomfortable during normal activity.

☐ **VISUALIZE ONE COMPLETE OUTFIT** Can you get dressed using this new item, including shoes? If not, skip it.

🕐 GOT 4 MINUTES?

Purchase with confidence

Before you buy from a store with a poor return policy, search Froogle .com. You may discover the same item at an online vendor with a better policy. Bonus: Your purchase will be delivered to your door.

⏱ GOT 10 MINUTES?
Be a savvy buyer
It's easy to find a bargain with these stylist tips for navigating the sales racks.

Score end-of-season deals. "Department stores start marking down fall/winter merchandise in January, and serious spring/summer markdowns happen in July," says Rebecca DiLiberto, style director of LivePersonalShoppers.com, a free online site. If you happen to be traveling in Western Europe, says Heather Kenny, a wardrobe consultant in Chicago, the government sets the sales, and they happen twice yearly (January/February and June/July).

Surf the stores. "You can brave the crowds in stores, but it's easier to scour department store websites for deals," DiLiberto says. It could be cheaper, too: She says online sales at, for example, Saks.com or Nordstrom.com are often better than those in the stores.

Make friends in the right places. Buddy up to that boutique saleswoman whose fashion sense you admire, and she may let you know ahead of time when sales will start and perhaps even put aside items in your size. "It's important to develop a relationship," says April Zdrilic-Shen, a style consultant in San Francisco and New York City. "That's a good way to get a head start on getting stuff before the general public."

Be in the know. Put yourself on as many store mailing lists as possible, both e-mail and snail mail. "You'll learn about the sales ahead of time, and you might even score a coupon for a discount," Kenny says.

⏱ GOT 15 MINUTES?
Make online shopping a cinch
Here's how to be sure you shop as successfully on the Web as you would in person.

1 **COMPARE PRICES** Search engines such as Shopzilla and Froogle scour thousands of online stores in seconds. Stay informed about markdowns with ShopItToMe.com. The free service scans different sites and e-mails you when your favorite styles go on sale.

2 **AWAKEN EARLY** Morning is when many sites post the latest merchandise. "We introduce at least 150 new styles every day at 6:31 A.M. The scary part is that often by 6:32 A.M., most of the good stuff has been snagged!" says Melissa Payner, president and CEO of Bluefly.

3 **SHOP FOR KEEPS** If you're between sizes, order both and send one back, Payner suggests. Reputable sites have lenient return policies and often free shipping.

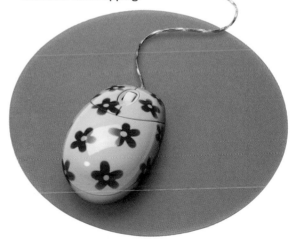

❋ ⏱ GOT 1 MINUTE? **Double up**
When you come upon shoes you adore, pick up a second pair before it vanishes from the market. The same rule applies to great-fitting jeans. Buy two pairs. Have one hemmed to wear with flats, and leave the other long to wear with heels. Indulgence never felt so smart.

🕐 GOT 10 MINUTES?
Get the most out of every outfit you own

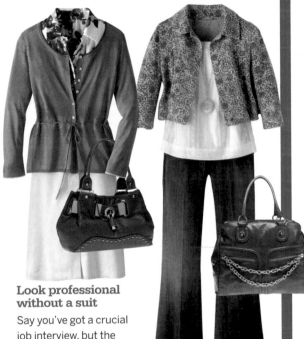

Look professional without a suit

Say you've got a crucial job interview, but the place you want to work isn't all that corporate. What do you wear? Chic your way to the top in a softer version of a suit by pulling together separates. As you would with a traditional suit, choose a patterned blouse so you're not a mass of solids, but go with a bold, not prissy, print to do away with any fussiness. Pair it with a structured skirt. In lieu of a jacket, a fine knit drapes nicely to give you polish. (No bulky cardigans!)

Make your office clothes work for the weekends

Closet stuck in 9 to 5? You can still create Saturday style. Pair the top half of a fave office outfit with denim to increase the casual factor, then mess things up a little: Leave your top untucked; push up jacket sleeves; layer necklaces. And carry that bright handbag you fear is too loud for work!

🕐 GOT 5 MINUTES?
Hide your straps!

A new tank top: sexy. Bra straps that show: not. Kendall Farr, author of *The Pocket Stylist* (Gotham), has this tip. On each strap of a tank, sew an inch-long ribbon with snaps on either end so it can cross under your bra strap and snap to the tank top. Now your bra is anchored to your top and won't peek out.

🕐 GOT 4 MINUTES?
Expand your wardrobe options

Artful layering can turn a few outfits into dozens. To get the look right, make your inner layer the longest and thinnest. Try a camisole under a cashmere V-neck. Then top that with something snug—a cropped jacket or, to reveal more of what's beneath, a nipped-in vest.

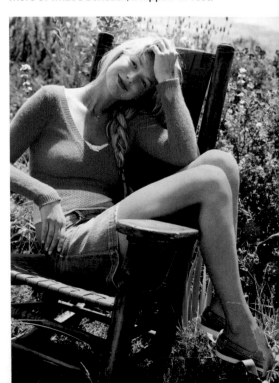

🕐 GOT 2 MINUTES? Select the right heel height

Flats? Stilettos? Kitten heels? Wedges? The proper heel makes you look put-together, say Emily Current and Meritt Elliott of the styling team Maude, whose clients include Mandy Moore and Fiona Apple. Their recommendations:

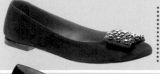

| | Flats | With ballet flats, structured dresses and trousers are Audrey Hepburn—adorable. Longer skirts look sexy with a little toe showing. Choose strappy sandals to draw the eye from the feet up bare legs to the hemline. |

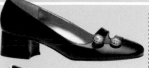

| | Midheight heels | Opt for a midheel (around 1½ inches) at work, when you don't want your shoes to stand out. They add height, helping your pants fall properly. |

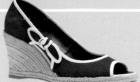

| | Platforms and wedges | Choose these fun shapes to increase height yet still stay comfortable. Wear them with high-waisted pants; tailored, to-the-knee shorts; and baby-doll dresses or 1960s-style ones that puff out at the waist. |

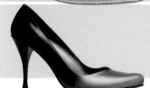

| | Stilettos | Your highest heels will be great with cocktail dresses, wide-legged trousers, pencil skirts and dresses, cigarette pants, even some jeans—in short, any silhouette that can handle a "look at me" shoe. |

🕐 GOT 3 MINUTES?
"Tailor" an outfit without sewing

● SELF's stylists swear by Topstick tape (WardrobeSupplies.com). The double-sided tape was designed to make toupees stay put, but it works great to temporarily refasten a sagging hem.
● Topstick can also prevent an R-rated moment if your dress has a plunging neckline. It can keep slipping straps in place, too. For better placement, attach the tape to the fabric first, then your body. For better stick, avoid moisturizing.

🕐 GOT 1 MINUTE?
Do away with deodorant streaks

Quickly get those embarrassing white marks off your shirt with a Gal Pal ($10; Gal-Pal.com), a reusable pink sponge that swipes off smudges almost instantly. SELF's in-house fashion experts give it an A+.

🕐 GOT 1 MINUTE?
Tame a zipper

Got a hard-to-reach zipper? Steal this idea from the design of wet suits, which have a long strap on the back zipper: Thread dental floss through the zipper's tab, bend over so the floss flops past your shoulder, grasp and pull. All set!

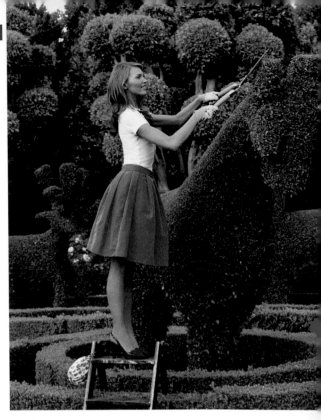

⏱ GOT 10 MINUTES?
Look longer and leaner

YOU DON'T NEED a "skinny mirror." These shape-flattering clothes will bring on compliments of the "You're so thin!" variety every time you wear them.

THREE-QUARTER-LENGTH SLEEVES hide thick upper arms, help your arms appear graceful and emphasize one of your most delicate features: your wrists.

BELL SLEEVES are another fab flab fighter. The flared cuff allows your biceps to look narrow in comparison.

LOW-WAISTED FLAT-FRONT TROUSERS are the fashion equivalent of The Abdomenizer because the straight no-nonsense cut holds in your midriff and the low waist camouflages width. Make them even more flattering: Remove the pockets. You don't need the additional fabric; even if it's satin, it creates unnecessary bulk in an area you may feel has enough on its own.

A-LINE SKIRTS lie close to your midsection then gently flare away from your hips and rear end to gracefully skim over any lumps and bumps.

V-NECK COLLARS or deeply unbuttoned blouses create a vertical line that makes your neck appear long, distracts from a double chin and draws attention to the center of your body for a slimmer appearance overall.

SLEEVELESS TOPS are controversial. Some women insist on covering not-so-taught triceps with a sleeve, any sleeve, even babyish cap sleeves. Big mistake. When you bare your arm shoulder to wrist with a sleeveless shirt, you create a long, lean line. A sleeve that ends at those troublesome triceps draws attention to them.

⏱ GOT 2 MINUTES?
Strike a slim pose

Are you convinced there's truth in that old chestnut "The camera adds 10 pounds"? Seem svelte in every picture with this what-to-wear tip from Victoria Will, a professional photographer in New York City: Wear bright colors on parts you want to show off. But beware of black: The visual void it creates can make your body seem bigger.

⏱ GOT 10 MINUTES?
Make sure everything in your closet is flattering

Banish these clothes and you'll never have to ask, "Do I look fat?"
- Raglan sleeves. You can root for the home team; just don't do it in a baseball tee. It makes shoulders appear rounder than they really are.
- Cap sleeves, short sleeves with elastic or ruffles and tight T-shirt sleeves that hit at your widest part can make your arms look heavier.
- Scoop necks add even more roundness up top to well-endowed gals.
- Pants that taper to the ankle create an upside-down pyramid that makes hips and thighs look heavy disproportionately to your calves.
- Pleated pants add bunched up fabric where you want it least.
- Ankle-strap shoes cut across your legs, stopping the eye and making calves look chunky. Only spindly legs that need heft look good in them.
- Vertical stripes aren't a slam dunk for slimming. In some cases they can pull or ripple on your body, creating unattractive curvy lines.

⏱ GOT 7 MINUTES?
Disguise your flaws Now you see it, now you don't. Solve any trouble spot with our custom figure-fixing chart.

IF YOU HAVE	THEN WEAR
Broad shoulders	Jackets with shoulder seams that hit right at the shoulder or even a bit closer to your neck. This cut creates a sparrowlike appearance. Conversely, shoulder pads make you look like a linebacker. Also, avoid boatneck tops, which make your neck seem wider than it is.
A large bust	A V-neck. You're probably thinking, won't that show too much? But a V-neck draws the eye up to your face so the focus isn't all on your chest. If you're too shy to show off that much skin, wear a shirt that buttons down the front and flip up the collar to create a more conservative V.
Thick arms	Bling! Sparkling jewelry on your wrists and fingers will make your limbs seem lithe and distract the eye from any jiggle.
A short waist	A top or dress with an Empire waist or, conversely, a tunic that skims your torso and ends somewhere in the hip region. In either case, by shifting your waistband, you're giving the illusion of a longer midsection.
A long waist	Pants with a relatively high rise—right below or at the belly button. They are ideal, but skirts with a high waistband work as well. Low rises add an unwanted inch or two to an already long torso.
Thick calves	Knee-length skirts. The idea is to expose as much of the calf as possible. This elongates the leg for a slimming effect.
Chunky thighs	Full-length boot-cut pants. A pant leg that's consistently sized from thigh to calf results in a long line.
Wide hips and butt	Wide-legged pants, which offset and deemphasize hips and thighs. Also, a low rise (the waist sits a finger or two below your belly button) keeps fabric from creeping over your midsection and creating even more pudge.
A pear shape	Tops in a substantial fabric and structured cut. They balance out a wider bottom half and create an hourglass. Flimsy fabrics like silk don't add enough volume up top.

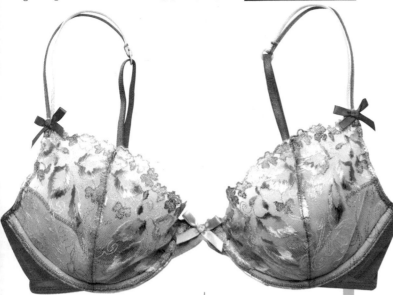

🕐 GOT 9 MINUTES?
Buy the best bra for you

THE RIGHT BRA can make you look 5 to 7 pounds thinner (and years younger), but finding it can be maddeningly difficult. The solution: a professional fitter. Go to a lingerie shop or department store and have one of the seasoned saleswomen find you a bra that works for your body. Here's a preview of what an appointment with your new breast friend will reveal.

Your size Amazingly, many women merely guess at their size and are stunned to learn from a fitter that they are not the 36D they believed but actually a 34C. Add in a 5- or 6-pound weight gain or loss, and you're a new size. Aren't you curious to find out what it is?

Your shape A fitter sees your breasts as a clock. In your bouncy 20s you may have been full on the outer edge of your breasts, around three and nine o'clock. Later, thanks to gravity, the passing of time or nursing, fullness may shift to a lower area, say around six o'clock. Similarly, when you're young a fitter might give you a side-seamed bra to mold nine o'clock breasts. Later, she'd offer a bra with an extra sling (a supportive layer of fabric under the lower part of the cup) to support your more experienced six o'clock breasts.

Your cleavage You know you've found the perfect fit when your bra "tacks" to your chest, meaning it lies snugly against your skin. If your bra isn't doing this right now, it's not the right bra. Get thee to a fitter!

🕐 GOT 10 MINUTES?
Round out your lingerie wardrobe

You have a drawerful of basic bras and panties, but sometimes basics aren't enough. These outfit-specific must-haves will make you look impeccably dressed, says Rebecca Apsan, owner of the lingerie store La Petite Coquette in New York City.

SEAMLESS CONTROL PANTIES Sure, thongs prevent panty lines, but they do nothing to smooth bumps and bulges under body-skimming skirts and dresses. These to-the-thigh skivvies are invisible and give you a smooth, slim line.

LASER-CUT PANTIES When you don't need bulge control but do want to prevent lines, you can still avoid the torturous thong. Laser-cut fabric edges don't fray, which eliminates the need for bumpy seams. A nude pair practically disappears under a pair of white pants.

T-SHIRT BRA It prevents noticeable nipples while going unseen under clingy sweaters, jersey fabrics and, yes, a T-shirt.

SILKY CAMISOLE A pretty, drapey version of the cami can be worn as a liner under sheer blouses, Apsan says, and as a way to dress up blazers and cardigans.

GOT 30 SECONDS?
Check a bra's life span
Purchase bras that fit when fastened on the loosest hook. When you have to use a tighter hook, your bra's elastic is giving way, and you should replaced it.

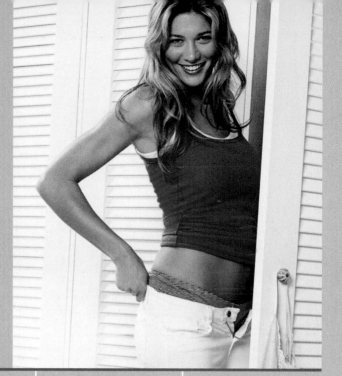

🕐 **GOT 4 MINUTES?**

Understand underwear

Undies shouldn't bind, crawl up or dig into any part of your body. Ideally, you wouldn't notice them at all (and certainly others shouldn't!). Pick the right style for any situation with these guidelines.

Bikinis

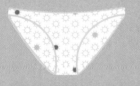

Full bikini panties work best for fit, lean women. For curvier and fuller shapes, string bikinis hide visible panty lines (VPL). For comfort, stick with cotton fabrics or seamless microfiber. Silk and satin bikinis are sexy but bunch up under clothes.

Thongs

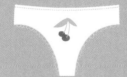

They help with VPL, but some gynecologists warn they are a back-to-front route for bacteria and can lead to health issues. Save them for tight skirts or pants with no back pockets, and choose wider-back butterfly-style thongs with a cotton crotch.

Boy shorts

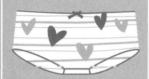

These are great with low-slung jeans or trousers. The hipster style skims the bottom of your derriere; full coverage versions are also available. Many men say they find this style sexier than a thong.

Briefs

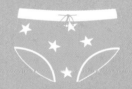

These comfortable full-coverage panties have a high waistline, which is why the brief shape is also common for body slimmers or shapers that control bulges. Spanx, Donna Karan's Body Perfect line and Assets at Target are great options.

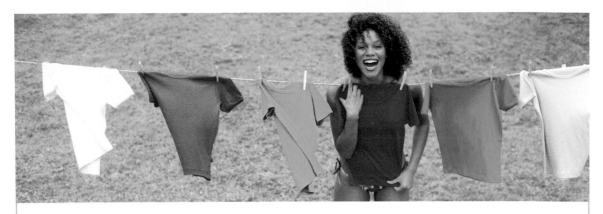

🕐 GOT 12 MINUTES?

Solve any stain Eradicate the most common stains with these tips from Alan Spielvogel of the National Cleaners Association in New York City.

STAIN	WHAT YOU SHOULD DO
Grease	Apply a citrus-based dishwashing liquid to the stain. Cover a spoon with a paper towel and tap the area; flush with cold water. Still stained? Mix 1 teaspoon laundry detergent, 2 ounces white vinegar and 2 ounces cold water. Apply to stain; rinse with cold water.
Red wine, coffee	Mix 2 ounces white vinegar, 2 ounces cold water and 1 teaspoon laundry detergent. Apply to stain and tap with a paper towel–covered spoon. Flush with cold water.
Lipstick	Sparingly apply petroleum jelly, then tap with a paper towel–covered spoon. Flush the area with lighter fluid or mineral spirits to dissolve the stain. Repeat if necessary. Blot the area with a dry towel or paper towel and leave in a well-ventilated place to dry.
Blood	Apply a solution of 1 teaspoon liquid laundry detergent, ½ teaspoon clear ammonia and 4 ounces cold water. Tap as above and repeat if necessary. Flush with cold water.
Ink	For ballpoint pens, follow the steps for lipstick. For rollerball ink stains (which contain water-based liquid), apply a citrus dishwashing liquid and tap with a with a paper towel–covered spoon; flush with cold water. If stain remains, use the procedure for red wine.

🕐 GOT 4 MINUTES?
Take salt marks off winter boots

Mix 1 tablespoon white vinegar with 1 cup water. Dip a cotton ball in the solution, gently wipe away the stain and set the boots aside to allow them to air-dry. If a snowy winter is predicted, keep the leftover solution for next time!

🕐 GOT 1 MINUTE?
Keep grease from staining

Stylists swear by baby powder to soak up oil. Dripped salad dressing on your lap? Sprinkle the spot as soon as possible, then pat, wipe and repeat.

⏱ GOT 3 MINUTES?
Learn to wash smarter

LAUNDERING YOUR FAVORITE wardrobe items properly will make them look newer and last longer, which saves you money. Use this fabric care guide from Linda Cobb of Phoenix, who is known as the Queen of Clean.

COTTON Machine wash light colors in warm water, brights that bleed in cold. Dry on low. Remove while still damp and iron immediately on the hot setting. Wash durable cottons such as T-shirts in hot water.
CASHMERE Dry-clean, or hand wash in cool water and a gentle soap for hand washables (like Woolite). Put a few drops of hair conditioner in the rinse water to soften the fabric. Roll in a towel to remove excess water. Dry flat.
LINEN Hand or machine wash linen in warm water. Iron while still damp, adding starch to prevent creasing. Use a hot iron on heavyweight linens, a warm iron on lighter-weight ones and blends of linen with other fibers.
WOOL Hand wash sweaters in cold water. Rinse several times; add a few drops of hair conditioner to the water to keep fibers soft. Blot with a towel and dry flat.

⏱ GOT 2 MINUTES?
Prevent blue jeans from fading

Dry-cleaning stops color loss, but the free method is to turn jeans inside out and wash on cold; hang to dry. (The dryer is as big a cause of fading as the washer.) Your denim's color will last for years.

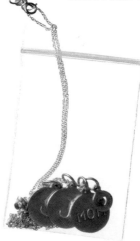

⏱ GOT 1 MINUTE?
Stop knots

If your necklaces tend to get tangled, store them in small ziplock bags with the clasp hanging out, advises Mandy Carol, production manager at Tenthousandthings, a boutique in New York City.

⏱ GOT 9 MINUTES? Squeeze more life out of your shoes

Your shoes endure a lot of punishment and keep on kicking. Here's what you (with the help of a trusted cobbler) can do to preserve them in the best condition.

Before you wear them

PLAY TAPS Have protective metal or rubber taps attached to your shoes' toe tips and heels, recommends style consultant April Zdrilic-Shen.

GET SOLE Thick rubber guards the bottoms of heavy winter shoes and boots but can spoil the lines of delicate footwear. For these, thin peel-and-stick soles (sold at the shoe repair shop) are a short-term solution. (You'll have to replace them every one or two outings.)

While you wear them

FEEL CUSHY Have a padded insole placed underneath part or all of the sock lining (the inside bottom of the shoe), advises Tony Pecorella, president of Modern Leather Goods Repair Shop in New York City. It adds to your comfort and won't noticeably change the fit of the shoe.

AVOID WEAR AND TEAR Keep an eye out for worn-down heels. Replace them at the first signs of wear. Wait too long, and your fave pair won't be easily repairable.

Before you store them

CLEAN UP Don't put a pair of shoes away right after a trek through the mud or snow. Wipe down soles with a damp paper towel and let dry. If the leather is stained, use a leather cleaner or conditioner, or get a pro polish.

PACK WITH CARE Storing shoes in plastic bags can trap moisture that leads to mildew. If the shoes came with a cloth bag, use that. Cloth allows leather to breathe. Stuff the tops of boots with tissue paper, or use boot trees.

🕐 GOT 12 MINUTES?

Pare down your closet painlessly Twice a year, wave farewell to tattered jeans, bid adieu to threadbare tees and rid your wardrobe of anything not in regular rotation. Suffer from fashion separation anxiety? Let this flowchart make the tough calls for you.

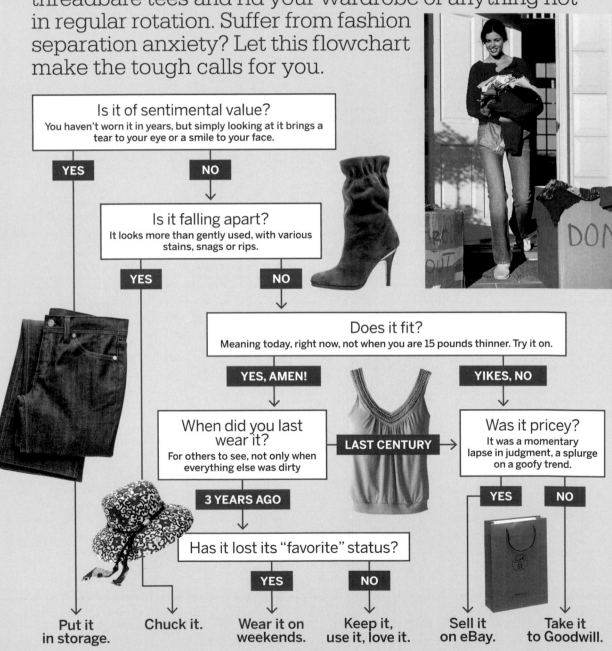

Is it of sentimental value?
You haven't worn it in years, but simply looking at it brings a tear to your eye or a smile to your face.

YES → NO →

Is it falling apart?
It looks more than gently used, with various stains, snags or rips.

YES → NO →

Does it fit?
Meaning today, right now, not when you are 15 pounds thinner. Try it on.

YES, AMEN! → YIKES, NO →

When did you last wear it?
For others to see, not only when everything else was dirty

LAST CENTURY →

Was it pricey?
It was a momentary lapse in judgment, a splurge on a goofy trend.

YES → NO →

3 YEARS AGO →

Has it lost its "favorite" status?

YES → NO →

Put it in storage.　Chuck it.　Wear it on weekends.　Keep it, use it, love it.　Sell it on eBay.　Take it to Goodwill.

GOT 30 SECONDS?
Spring-clean efficiently
Before tackling the closet, line up four boxes for: (1) off-season clothes, (2) things to donate or sell, (3) items to repair and (4) trash. You won't be left with a mess.

GOT 2 MINUTES?
Save your clothes

Store your own mini cleaning kit in your closet so your clothing will look sharper longer. Include:

A LINT BRUSH When your pet has a thick coat of hair, it's gorgeous. When you have a thick coat of your pet's hair...it's not so gorgeous.

SCISSORS Having some handy keeps you from ripping off tags with your hands and risking holes.

A TINY TRASH CAN Toss in your tags, plus the crumpled receipts and movie stubs you find in your pockets.

STAIN STICKERS Ask your dry cleaner to share some with you so you can mark dirty spots as you undress.

GOT 15 MINUTES?
Get dressed in a jiff

1 **HANG** everyday duds in the middle of your closet, bookended by layers on the left (sweaters, jackets) and fancy clothes on the right (sequined tops, dressy skirts). "That way you can see all your favorite clothes front and center, making them easier to choose from," says SELF fashion director Evyan Metzner. "Then you can grab from either side to add a little warmth or accent."

2 **USE** a hanging sweater bag for your workout clothes. "You can organize by day," says Mary Mobley of Spaceworks NY in New York City. Place everything you need, including socks and sports bras, in one compartment so each morning you can grab fresh gear and go.

3 **STASH** accessories such as gloves, scarves, totes and umbrellas—the indispensable items you reach for last as you're walking out the door—in an over-the-door shoe-storage unit with clear plastic pouches.

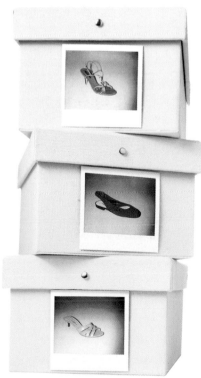

GOT 8 MINUTES?
Find your shoes fast

Maximize closet floor space: Line up your frequently worn pairs of shoes, alternating toe-in, toe out, says Meryl Starr of Let's Get Organized! in LaGrangeville, New York. Place out-of-season pairs in boxes bearing photos of what's inside. No camera? Write a full description on the box—"brown, low-heeled sandals with tan straps." Stow the boxes under the bed.

⏱ GOT 5 MINUTES?

Tie one on String bikinis are a summer showstopper. To avoid revealing *too* much, use these clever tips from SELF's fashion editors.

- To gauge how tightly to tie the strings on each side, lay the bottom over a pair of your underwear.
- Wet the strings before tying. Damp fabric stretches, which is why your suit sags when you come out after a dip.
- If you don't like the bulge of a bow under a sarong, simply tie a knot and let the strings hang—a sexy look in itself.
- Don't be afraid to snip the strings if they're too long. Now you can dive in with total confidence.

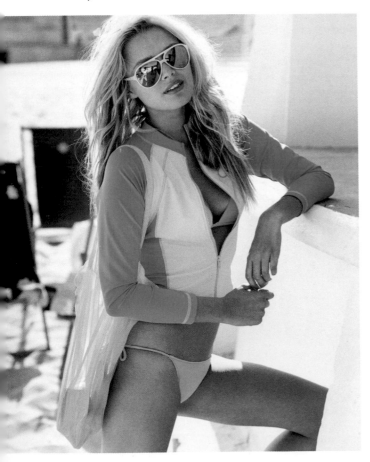

⏱ GOT 4 MINUTES?

Soup up your sarong

Tie your favorite sarong into shapes that show off your best body parts.

IF YOU LOVE YOUR	WEAR IT AS A
Legs »	**Mini tube dress** Fold it lengthwise and hold it behind you, bringing the sides around your chest and knotting in front so ends drape down.
Abs »	**Long skirt** Wrap it around your hips and tie it in the center of your waist, creating a low V. The slanted angle is super flattering.
Arms »	**Halter dress** Open it full length behind your back and wrap it around you, crisscrossing the ends and tying behind your neck.

⏱ GOT 15 MINUTES?

Shield your eyes

Your celebrity-chic shades turn heads. But do they also harm your eyes? These days, most pairs do block UV rays, but if you're unsure, have an optician or optometrist check (dark lenses prove nothing). If not, she can apply a protective coating.

GOT 12 MINUTES?

Spot a feel-sexy swimsuit

There's a confidence-boosting, strutworthy suit for every body type. Prepare to rule the pool!

IF YOU ARE	LOOK FOR
Bottom-heavy	A dark bottom and a lighter top. Those often-recommended slimmers draw the eye up and away from trouble zones. In a one-piece, look for a straight neckline (a strapless suit works well) to broaden shoulders, balancing you out.
Top-heavy	A suit in your exact cup size and with a triple hook closure so the top fits (no spillover) and supports (no sag) as well as a bra would. Bows tied at the hips fool the eye into seeing an hourglass shape, not an inverted pyramid.
Petite	A two-piece, preferably with a bikini bottom, not the higher-waisted brief style. The bare stretch of skin elongates your torso. Avoid ties on the bottom, which draw attention to short legs. Choose high leg cutouts for a longer line.
Round in the tummy	A high-waisted brief and a long tankini top. The pieces should slightly overlap for maximum control. Suits made with extra Lycra suck you in. A bold print will keep the eye traveling instead of resting on trouble spots.
Long-waisted	Horizontal stripes to offset the length of your midsection. (Not a stripes lover? A contrasting waistband on the bottom and chestband on the top achieve the same effect.) A high-waisted bottom helps shorten your torso.
Small-busted	Thin, molded cups to encourage a subtle, natural-looking swell. (You're trying to enhance what you've got, not pretend two lumps of foam are your breasts.) A behind-the-neck tie or a halter top will pull you up and in.
Plus-sized	A strapless one-piece to camouflage likely trouble spots and showcase pretty shoulders. Don't feel wed to a solid color. Yes, that slims, but a pattern above the waist or as trim at the top lends definition and keeps the eye moving.

GOT
6 MINUTES?

Baby that bathing suit

To counteract saltwater and chlorine, try this tip from Lisa Curran, a swimwear designer in NYC: After each wearing, soak your suit for four minutes in cool water with 1 teaspoon Cetaphil facial cleanser and a sprig of fresh mint, then rinse.

GOT
2 MINUTES?

Say good-bye to blisters

Make stiff new leather sandals softer: Wet a cotton pad with rubbing alcohol and swipe it across the straps, inside and out (only once, to avoid drying out the leather). Wear the sandals around the house. Alcohol speeds the natural stretching process.

GOT
2 MINUTES?

Help ward off sunburn

To be sure your T-shirt offers some sun protection, hold it up to a window. Tightly woven dark fabrics let in less light and protect better than loose-weave pale ones. But even if it's black and as thick as armor, don't skip the sunscreen!

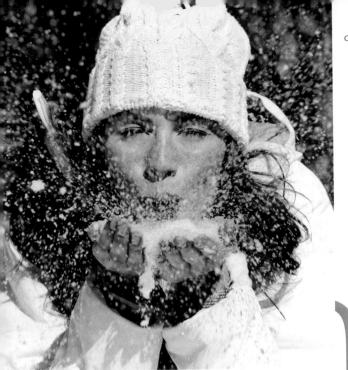

⏱ GOT 7 MINUTES?
Be warm in *brrr* weather

"JUST BECAUSE it's cold out, you don't have to look like Frosty the Snowman," says celebrity stylist Nick Steele, who has dressed Beyoncé, Katie Couric and Claire Danes. To stay cozy but chic, he recommends...

1 Start with a great foundation. Silk long underwear keeps you toasty without adding unwanted bulk. Bonus: Unlike cotton, silk wicks away moisture.

2 Get a coat with an inside zipper and a button closure over that. This pairing provides two layers of warmth. Go with a deep hood or one that cinches closed to keep body heat from escaping through your head.

3 Add an extra layer to shed. Invest in a "technical" fleece jacket for under your coat. Find one in the skiing or snowboarding section at a sporting goods store. A dressier option: a cashmere hoodie.

4 Choose gloves that have elastic or straps that tighten at the wrist to keep out the cold. Pick ones that are lined and have a waterproof exterior.

5 For bone-chilling temperatures, get the secret weapon professional skiers and Hollywood actresses use. Purchase one-use hand and foot warmers that fit in pockets or shoes and keep you warm for hours. You can find them at sporting goods stores.

⏱ GOT 10 MINUTES?
Buy the right winter boots
Follow the checklist below so your tootsies survive the season.

- For a versatile pair, pick a dark, neutral color such as brown. Good news: It will also hide stains.
- A stacked wedge provides some support so you can maintain your balance in uneven terrain. Rubber soles prevent slips and skids.
- Tall boots that fold down are like two pairs in one. Wear them high when you need warmth, folded over once you get to the office.
- Choose waterproof suede; it's as durable as it is chic. Treat all boots with a protective spray before braving the elements.
- Look for a shearling or faux-fur lining. Both keep feet comfy and warm and add a trendy touch.

⏱ GOT 5 MINUTES?
Replace a lost trench coat belt

You lost the belt to your trench. What do you do? See it as an opportunity to give your coat more style! A jeweled tie belt wraps easily, and the touch of glitter makes a basic coat special. Or toughen up your trench with a mock-croc belt. Measure before you buy, though—the belt should go through the loops, not over them.

⏱ GOT 4 MINUTES?
Know the most common chilly-climate fabrics

Cashmere The fine, soft, downy undercoat of the Kashmir goat from India, Pakistan and nearby countries makes a silky, strong fiber that gains durability when it's mixed with wool or other materials. Extremely soft and warm, but can be pricey if thick.

Down The supersoft feathers that grow beneath the upper feathers of ducks, geese and other waterfowl are extremely warm when used as a filling in outdoor wear. The drawback? Down may cause allergies and, when it gets wet, smells like damp dog and takes a while to dry. One solution: Substitute a garment made with warm, wicking synthetic down (check the tag).

Fleece This warm, durable, light, breathable, stretchy, soft and washable fabric is made from polyethylene terephthalate, a synthetic material also used to make soda bottles. It's comfortable against your skin, dries easily if you get wet and, unlike some natural fibers, better versions won't pill even after multiple washes.

Wicking synthetics Synthetics are your friend in winter, especially for outdoor gear. They are designed to pull moisture away from your skin, preventing chapping, and can be comfortably layered. Names to know: Therma Fleece, Drylete, Dri-Fit, UltraSensor (all of which are combined with stretchy spandex) and Coolmax.

Wool This fiber sheared from sheep is strong and an excellent insulator. It contains the natural oil lanolin, which may cause allergies. Other disadvantages are a tendency to shrink and to be a tasty treat to moths.

⏱ GOT 12 MINUTES? Sift through the coat rack in a snap
Consult this chart to pinpoint the perfect coat for any occasion.

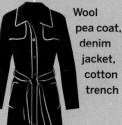

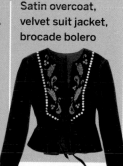

	FABRIC	COLOR	EMBELLISHMENT	LENGTH AND FIT	3 MUST-HAVES
Casual	Stiffer, heavier materials are practical and can stand up to everyday wear and tear. You can't go wrong with wool, tweed, leather, corduroy or denim.	Steer clear of busy patterns; a casual coat should go with nearly everything in your closet. Select a warm neutral, such as olive, navy, brown or burgundy.	Don't overdo the details. On a basic coat, small touches—such as contrasting stitching, toggle closures, a hood or a belt—are all the adornment you need.	Wear a thin T-shirt under a thick sweater when you shop to be sure it fits well over both.	Wool pea coat, denim jacket, cotton trench
Dressy	Sumptuous textures convey luxury and polish. Try velvet (lined for warmth), faux fur or a cashmere blend, or anything with a lustrous finish, such as silk or satin.	Of course, classic black is chic and timeless. Feeling adventurous? Deep plum or any type of metallic will match everything and add a splash of personality.	Closures should be subtle; dainty hooks or small buttons achieve the right effect. Have fun with feminine touches like three-quarter sleeves or a bright satin lining.	A bulky cut looks wrong for evening. If you're wearing a cocktail dress, choose a tailored, streamlined coat that hits roughly between the knee and midcalf.	Satin overcoat, velvet suit jacket, brocade bolero

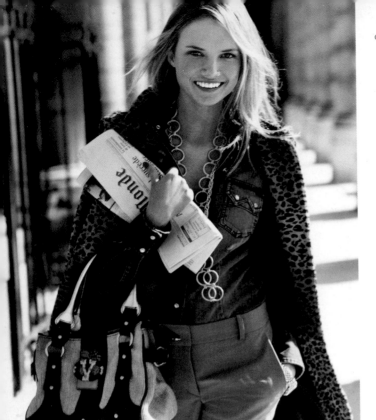

🕐 GOT 6 MINUTES?
Bling it on!

Your clothes aren't the only wardrobe items that can help enhance your shape.

1 Layer several long chain necklaces over a turtleneck and your torso will seem longer, which makes you appear taller.

2 Chandelier earrings add glitz. If your neck is short, choose a light color so they recede yet bring sparkle to your face.

3 Round-faced? Get earrings that hang right below chin level. They elongate your face much as vertical stripes do your body.

🕐 GOT 12 MINUTES?
Complete your shoe collection

THE THREE PAIRS of shoes no well-heeled woman should be without:

D'ORSAY PUMP The pointy toe, high heel and extremely low profile on the sides create a sexy line and make calves look lean.

V-THROAT SHOE This shoe is like a V-neck for your foot, making it look longer by drawing attention to your toes and giving your ankle a more delicate appearance.

LOW-CUT MULES This easy-to-wear style won't break up the line of your leg and gives you an overall ladylike air.

🕐 GOT 1 MINUTE?
Screen your bag

Hoisting a hefty tote can lead to back pain, neck strain and headaches, notes sports medicine expert and SELF contributing editor Lisa Callahan, M.D. Need to lighten up? Check all that apply.

☐ You carry both a purse and a tote bag.

☐ Your bag leaves an indentation and/or a red mark on your shoulder.

☐ After standing and holding your bag for five minutes, you long to put it down.

☐ You feel sore Tuesday morning after carrying your bag to work on Monday.

☐ When you hand your purse to a friend, she asks, "Is this a handbag or a sandbag?!"

Checked three or more? It's time to jettison that hardcover copy of *Anna Karenina.* Your back will thank you.

🕐 GOT 2 MINUTES?
Make a scarf chic

Look elegant, not soccer mom, with ideas from Renee Klein and Zoe Schaeffer, co-owners of the boutique Presse in Los Angeles.

● Create a scarf bracelet on your wrist; it's a little rock-and-roll, but with an elegant twist.

● Tie it to a strap on your handbag to add a dash of color and a little flutter.

● Wrap it around your head à la Jackie O. It should rest right over your hairline.

YOUR STYLE TO-DON'T LIST

»Don't get cold feet. Wear warm boots to and from the office, and stash loafers or cute pumps at your desk.

»Don't pack up your summer tees. Layer them for warmth and comfort.

»Don't be afraid to approach any salesperson, regardless of how snobby she seems. After all, it's her *job* to help you. By the same token, don't be afraid to refuse help if she hovers.

»Don't keep more than one pair of skinny jeans. One is a motivator. Two are a delusion. Love your size now.

»Don't be tempted to forgo your personal style by any fashion trend. What's truly "in" is being yourself.

»Don't worry if you misplace your umbrella. Consider it an excuse to buy yourself a new one in a cheery shade.

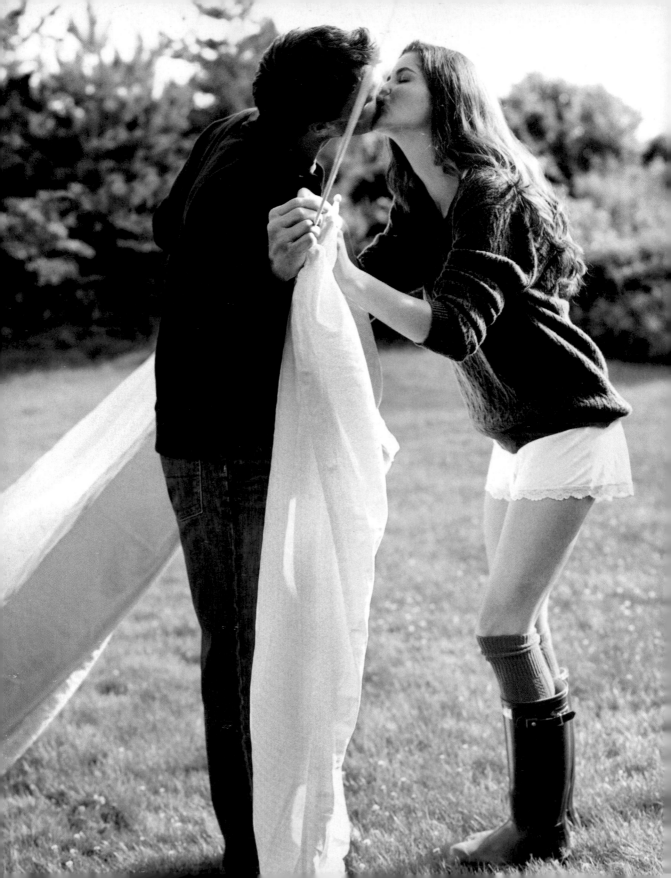

SPEEDY
sex
satisfiers

Ready? Set? Reconnect! Whether your relationship is only a few months old or you recently celebrated a double-digit anniversary, the following pages offer simple strategies to bring electrifying energy to your bedroom—or wherever else you're having sex. So get excited. You're merely moments away from watching your love life go from good to knock-your-socks-off incredible.

The only 10 things you need to know to have a happy, healthy, fulfilling sex life

This goes here. That goes there. Move this way. Actually, now a bit more that way. That's it! Sighs all around. And that concludes another night of gratifying sex. Regardless of what kind of sex you're having, it can usually be better. Memorize and practice (and practice) the following principles. You—and your partner—will thank us tonight!

1 Make sex a priority

Approach sex with the same diligence you bring to mundane tasks such as paying the electric bill. If you didn't do it, your lights would go out. If you ignore sex, well, your lights will go out in a figurative sense: You won't get the rejuvenating effects a good romp can have on your body and your relationship. Let's be honest. You do have time for sex—you've just been spending it on something else. Try choosing sex over doing laundry. It doesn't have to be an epic event. The more you have it, the less you need to make up for times you deferred. Plus, frequent sex takes pressure off. Instead of a tribute to your love, it can be merely fun!

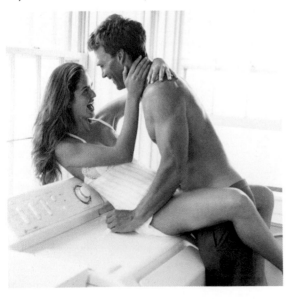

2 Practice equals pleasure

It may take two to tango, but it requires only one (and that would be you) to make your sex drive soar. "Masturbation lets you know what your body is capable of and prepares you to share that with your partner," says Pepper Schwartz, Ph.D., sociology professor at the University of Washington at Seattle. Regular stimulation keeps blood flowing to your genitals, which improves lubrication and sensation, making orgasms with your mate easier to achieve. Once you've mastered the turn-on yourself, you can't help but dive into bed with a partner. In one SELF survey, 22 percent of women who had sex five times a week also masturbated more than five times a week. "Women who masturbate regularly don't have less partnered sex; they actually have more," says Rachel Carlton Abrams, M.D., a women's health specialist in Santa Cruz, California. "It puts sex on the brain. When you think about it, you're more likely to act on it."

3 Talk the talk

There's no way around it: You need to tell your partner how to please you and determine what excites him, too. Start the conversation by asking what your mate likes with a few simple questions. Does this feel good? Is that better? Then invite him to ask you. Don't confine your chat to the bedroom either. It may be easier to talk over dinner. "As this back-and-forth becomes part of your ritual, you'll both feel comfortable describing what you want in detail," says Shannon Mullen, who runs sex-ed salons in New York City.

4 Find the right birth control for you

Nothing promotes a healthy sex life like being confident in your birth control. If you don't trust your method, switch ASAP. Nearly 60 percent of women say the right choice—one that lets them feel secure in bed—makes it easier to relax into the mood, reports the National Association of Nurse Practitioners in Women's Health in Washington, D.C. For effective options, see "Pick the Best Birth Control for You" (page 174).

5 Start moving!

Exercise and orgasm go hand in hand. Here's why: Cardio eases stress, revs energy and ups blood flow down south. Yoga and pilates bolster pelvic-floor muscles, which can intensify orgasms, and lifting weights stimulates testosterone, the hormone of arousal. Looking and feeling toned (any type of exercise helps) boosts body image. And if you work out pre-romp, your body releases adrenaline, which gives you in-the-mood momentum.

6 Pay attention

It's easy to have sex on autopilot. If you always do it in the dark, in the same position on the same bed, you're apt to tune out. You know what's coming, so your mind may wander rather than enjoy the feel of your partner's body, the smell of his neck, the sound of his breathing. Try a new position or a sexy video for inspiration. Changing just one aspect stirs your senses and sets a seductive mood. It also tells your lover he's special, which can make you feel close.

7 Reveal your fantasies

Sex is not only about your body. Your brain is involved, too. In a SELF survey, women who made love five times a week were more likely to think about it outside the bedroom. Got fantasies? Share them with your partner, then ask to hear his. Nothing says bonding like divulging your most private thoughts. Foreplay is a built-in bonus: After disclosing, you'll want to rip off each other's clothes.

8 Keep it safe

Herpes, syphilis, gonorrhea— you see these words in pamphlets at your doctor's office, but they have nothing to do with you, right? You can't be sure. The American Social Health Association in Research Triangle Park, North Carolina, estimates that more than half of all people will have an STD at some point in their life. (The United States has about 19 million new cases of STDs, including HIV, a year.) You don't have to abstain, but you do have to realize that there's a chance of infection. Ideally, you and your partner should get tested before sex. Until you know the score, be sure to use protection.

9 Forsake the fake

One of the biggest barriers to earth-shattering sex is the faux O. Why? Lying is intimacy's worst enemy. The message you're sending your lover is "You rock my world," when you're really thinking, Zzz. It's normal not to climax on occasion. But pretending you did robs you of a chance to be honest. On the flip side, letting your partner know you didn't get off—and that you're OK with it (if you are)—builds trust, shows you don't expect perfection and stymies resentment. Communication is key to an intimate sex life.

10 Celebrate yourself

Eighty-eight percent of women say "feeling fat" dulls their good time, and 71 percent fret that their partner won't like what he sees when they're naked, reports a SELF survey. Challenge your inner insults by reframing them in a more positive way. Rather than berating your butt, say, "My booty is muscular and strong." Sometimes, feeling body-proud takes practice. But once you feel it, you'll start enjoying sex more than you ever knew was possible.

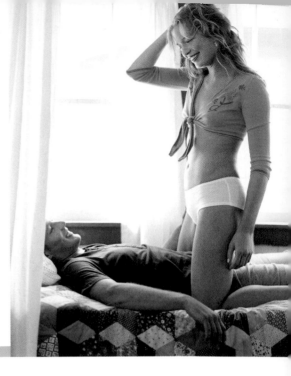

◕ GOT 7 MINUTES?
Identify (and solve!) sneaky sex saboteurs

If you're fairly certain the reason you're having ho-hum sex has more to do with your partner than you, your options are pretty simple: Speak up or trade up. But if you suspect that *you* may be getting in the way of your own satisfaction, the following solutions to those nagging roll-in-the-hay roadblocks should bolster your ability to bring that lovin' feeling back into the bedroom.

1 TOO TIRED TO GET IT ON?
You've had a long, stressful day, and your libido is in deep freeze. Or so you think. Truth is, you can get worked up simply by being responsive to your partner's advances even when you're not in the mood, says Michele Weiner-Davis, a social worker in Boulder, Colorado. "You might surprise yourself."

2 CAN'T RELAX?
Many women imagine their body will tell them when they want sex, but in fact, most of us need to set the stage: Unplug the phone, click off the news and worry about it tomorrow—whatever "it" is.

3 TAKE FOREVER TO CLIMAX?
You're the only one who cares. Most men, you'll find, are in absolutely no hurry to stop having sex. So relax—letting go of the goal and enjoying the experience might make it happen faster, says Laura Berman, Ph.D., director of the Berman Center, a mind/body clinic for women's sexual health in Chicago.

4 AFRAID TO SAY NO?
There's a distinction between having sex when you're not gung ho and gritting your teeth through it. If you're in a neutral zone, you can say, "Let's try it," and see if the fireworks start. If they don't or you don't feel like trying, speak up, "Sorry, how about tomorrow?"

5 IGNORING YOUR DESIRES?
Ever hear the expression "Help others by helping yourself"? It applies to sex, too. "If you tell him what you want, you'll be giving him what he needs," says relationship guru Drew Pinsky, M.D., of Los Angeles.

6 EMBARRASSED TO SAY WHAT YOU WANT?
Start off small ("Mmm, a bit to the left") and take it from there. He'd give anything to know what he can do to make you happy in bed. And if he wouldn't, he's the one who should be feeling embarrassed.

7 CRAVING A NEW POSITION?
If you always rely on the same-old go-to stance such as missionary, test-drive some new techniques. For ideas, delve into your fantasies or ask your partner what he might like to try. Still need some inspiration? Thumb through an illustrated how-to manual such as *The Guide To Getting It On* (Goofy Foot Press).

GOT 30 SECONDS?
Designate a driver
Seventy-two percent of couples who trade off initiating sex have orgasms all or most of the time, a SELF survey finds. Propose sex one week; let him do so the next.

⏱ GOT 5 MINUTES? Learn how to open up about lovemaking

Many women—even those raised on Madonna and *Sex and the City*—find it hard to make their desires understood. Fortunately, SELF is here to help with five common sexual communication problems. Try these tips tonight, and the only words you'll need between the sheets will be "Wow, that was fabulous!"

What you'd like to say	The subtle method	A more direct approach	Hit him over the head
"Try something new to get me in the mood. The massage and music I once hinted at were only examples!"	Go to a video for new ideas. Fast-forward to a sexy scene in a movie and comment on how fun it looks.	Buy him a how-to book that brims with fresh ways to get you going. Avoid titles with the word *idiot*.	Spell it out. The next time he puts on Sade again, say, "The music is nice, but I'd love to hear [fill in the blank]."
"Sex is always sweet, which is great, but every once in a while, I would love it if you totally took charge."	Share a dream you had in which he was more caveman than Casanova. He might have the same desire.	Leave something fun (a scarf or eye shades) on the bed. Suggest you try one during sex. Let him choose which.	Take him to a nearby sex toy store and point out the tiger-striped loincloth that turns you on.
"I want to start using a vibrator during sex, but that doesn't mean you're not good at what you do."	Buy a back massager. After he works on your back, point him to another area and ask, "How about there?"	Buy a mini-vibrator and include it in a basket of sexy goodies, so the focus isn't on the vibrator.	Ask him to buy a vibrator for you. Once he sees how much you like it, he'll want to share in the fun.
"I don't always have to have an orgasm. The sex is still good, even if it doesn't end with a bang."	To a goal-focused guy, sex minus an orgasm doesn't compute. To avoid scrutiny, keep the focus on him.	Ask him to do other ecstasy-provoking deeds for you, such as massaging your feet or your back.	Tell him you want to have sex but might not always climax and it's no big deal. You'll both enjoy it guilt-free.
"Quit channel surfing! If I'm really enjoying something that you're doing to me, don't keep switching it up."	Make an intense moaning sound. You can even add, "I love exactly what you're doing right now!"	Slowly but surely guide his hand back to the precise spot where you want it. He'll definitely get the hint.	In a sexy whisper, tell him that you prefer a certain speed or pressure when you're close to the finish line.

🕐 **GOT 1 MINUTE?**

Pinpoint potential libido killers

Hate what you see in the mirror? Don't! According to the *Journal of Sex Research,* a poor body image can sap sexual desire even more than entering menopause. If four or more of these scenarios ring true to you, hostile feelings about your body could be impeding your love of sex. Realizing their existence can help you begin to retrain your brain to be more positive.

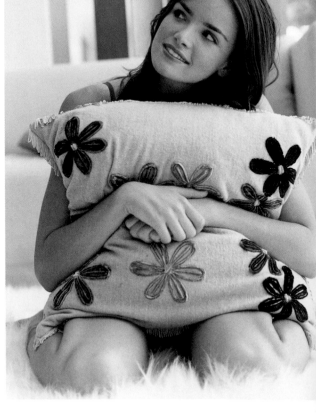

1 Your pal compliments you on your fabulous new wrap dress. Your reaction: "Yeah, right. This fabric totally shows off my love handles."

2 Whether you're doing loads of laundry or walking your dog, negative thoughts about your body nag you.

3 You have a tendency to refer to yourself as fat, flabby, gross, out of shape or ugly. You rarely think, I look good!

4 At the gym, you compare yourself with others. ("I'm thinner than she is, but my arms are more jiggly.")

5 You think that if only you could hit your goal weight, your life would instantly improve.

6 When you shop for new clothes, you often end up buying items that camouflage your figure.

7 You view your thin friends as prettier, more successful and happier than you.

8 Every day you ask someone to reassure you that you look OK.

9 You zero in on individual body parts in the mirror (your butt, thighs and chin) rather than assessing the whole picture.

✳ Need some body love? Focus on your positives: a great smile, strong legs, etc. Instant lift!

GOT 30 SECONDS?

Crank the stereo
Sixty-three percent of women say their fear of being seen or heard having sex is inhibiting. Put on a tune with a long, slow groove, and get down.

⏱ GOT 11 MINUTES?
Give your partner a pat on the back

YOU'RE NOT THE ONLY ONE whose sexual confidence sags on occasion. Chances are, your honey has moments when his lovemaking mojo requires some care and feeding—preferably from you. "Each partner needs to feel like the other person is in their corner," says Aline Zoldbrod, Ph.D., a psychologist in Lexington, Massachusetts. "Sex can be a huge way for couples to connect, but it doesn't happen in a vacuum." To rev his esteem—and your sex life—try these strategies.

MAKE A VOW to reach out to your beau every day, whether being sure to greet him (preferably with a kiss) or saying "I love you" out of the blue. Keep it up and both of you will feel closer and more loved.

REMIND YOURSELF that men often use sex as a way to feel cared for, whereas women tend to rely on words. "That's why he may initiate sex when you haven't spoken all day and be hurt when you say no," Zoldbrod explains. "Relationships need both sex and talk."

TREAT YOUR PARTNER like a child. No, we're not suggesting mothering him, but that you pay attention to him (ask about his day, for starters) and show him some affection. "Most women don't treat their mate half as well as they do their kids," Zoldbrod says.

REMINISCE by thinking of three nice things that drew you to your partner in the first place; ask him to reciprocate, then compare notes, Zoldbrod says. "Share them before sex; you'll feel better about your mate and yourself, which is bound to lead to a stronger connection."

⏱ GOT 3 MINUTES?
Forget feeling fat

The next time you're in a video store, slip into the adults-only section, if only for a moment. Chances are, you'll notice movies featuring all sorts of women: big-chested mamas, flat-chested waifs, scrawny butts, round butts, you name it. It's a good, quick reminder that men are turned on by all sorts of body types—including the curvy, juicy, fleshy bodies that many women spend so much time hating. Hey, the proof is in the porn.

⏱ GOT 1 MINUTE?
Make your sex life brighter

He likes the lights on, but you say no way? Skip the unflattering overhead glare and turn on a small table lamp instead. The diffuse light creates complimentary shadows that play up features, says Kenneth Wajda, a photographer in Westcliffe, Colorado. Not to mention that the warm glow is much more romantic.

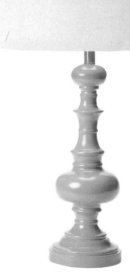

GOT 10 MINUTES?

Pick the best birth control for you Good sex is
love without fear of getting pregnant, if you want to avoid

Method	Success rate*	How it works
CONDOM	97%	A latex condom forms a barrier that traps and isolates sperm, keeping it (and STDs) away from your body.
DEPO-PROVERA	99%	Your doctor gives you a shot of progestin four times a year to inhibit ovulation and thicker cervical mucus.
DIAPHRAGM	94%	You coat a latex or silicone cup with spermicide and put it into the vagina to stop sperm's entry into the cervix.
FEMALE STERILIZATION	99%	The fallopian tubes are cut, blocked or sealed with heat; it can be done surgically or by inserting coils vaginally.
IMPLANON	99%	An implant, placed in the arm via a small incision, releases progestin to stop ovulation and menstruation.
IUD	99%	Intrauterine devices prevent pregnancy by interfering with fertilization, although doctors aren't sure how.
LYBREL	98% to 99%	This pill is taken 365 days a year, without placebo or break in pill time, completely eliminating your period.
NATURAL BIRTH CONTROL	Up to 95%	You use protection or abstain when you're most fertile, which you determine, in part, by checking cervical mucus.
NUVARING	99%	Worn 21 days a month, the vaginal ring releases hormones to block ovulation. Upon removal, you get a period.
ORTHO EVRA (THE PATCH)	99%	The same hormones typically found in the Pill are administered via a skin patch that is changed monthly.
THE PILL	99%	Oral contraceptives stop ovulation by altering hormone levels. Most popular method among women under 35.
SEASONALE	99%	You take this pill continuously for three months at a time, so you menstruate only four times a year.
THE TODAY SPONGE	About 90%	The soft foam disk blocks sperm's passage and dispenses spermicide at the same time.
VASECTOMY	99%	The tube that transports a man's sperm is surgically cut, cauterized or tied during the 30-minute procedure.
EMERGENCY OPTION PLAN B	89% when taken within 72 hours of sex	Plan B, aka the morning-after pill, prevents pregnancy by suppressing ovulation or preventing implantation.

uninhibited sex, and that's making it. The most common options:

Antipregnancy plus	Pitfalls
The man wears the birth control for a change.	You must use them consistently, and some contain the spermicide nonoxynol-9, which can cause irritation.
You deal with contraception only every three months, and you may have lighter periods.	Depo decreases estrogen and may lead to bone loss, so recommended use is limited to two years.
No hormones; use only when needed; not costly (about $45); lasts up to two years.	The spermicide may irritate; the device also presses against your urethra and may up your risk for urinary tract infections.
It's forever, baby.	It's forever, baby. Also, the nonsurgical coils (brand name Essure) take three months to become effective.
Implanon works for up to three years. Periods resume a month after removal.	Breakthrough bleeding can occur. There can also be tenderness at the incision site as well as a tiny scar.
Hormone-releasing Mirena protects for up to 5 years; copper ParaGard works for 10.	Some ParaGard users experience longer, heavier periods initially, and some Mirena users report acne.
No periods all year!	You can have unscheduled spotting at first. With no period, you might not know if you accidentally become pregnant.
It's natural, no Rx is needed and it's free.	Your fertility window could be up to a third of the month. Miscalculate and you might be shopping for maternity wear.
The steady hormone levels can mean few side effects such as headaches and nausea.	You have to keep track of when to insert and remove it. If you smoke, using NuvaRing can lead to heart problems.
You get a continuous release of hormones; it's as easy to use as a bandage.	It is visible and may cause skin irritation. One study found that it may be twice as likely as the Pill to cause blood clots.
More predictable periods and a lowered risk for ovarian and endometrial cancers.	You need to take it every day, and side effects may include nausea, headaches, breast tenderness and decreased libido.
Four periods a year!	You have to take it every day, and possible side effects include nausea, weight gain and breakthrough bleeding.
You insert it in advance of sex, and it requires no doctor's visit or prescription.	You have to keep the sponge in place for at least six hours following sex, and the spermicide may be irritating.
Uninhibited sex means your partner can focus on you; reversal is often possible.	Some pain and swelling may follow the procedure; you must use a backup method until sterilization is confirmed.
Condom broke? Forgot to take your pill? Had unprotected sex? There is a backup option.	An Rx isn't required if you're 18 or older, but drugstores keep Plan B behind the counter, so you have to ask for it.

*Success rates are based on using each method exactly as instructed. Each option helps prevent pregnancy, but only condoms help prevent STDs.

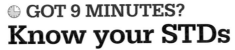

🕐 GOT 9 MINUTES?
Know your STDs

Wait, keep reading! It may not be your favorite topic, but learning about sexually transmitted diseases can improve your sex life. How? Feeling confident that you're fully protected can help you relax and enjoy sex. So check out the risks as well as how to identify and treat different types. It will make it that much easier to reach for the condoms every time you're ready for action.

Name	Symptoms	Dangers	Treatment
BACTERIAL			
Chlamydia	Often asymptomatic; may cause pain during urination, abnormal vaginal discharge or bleeding	Can lead to pelvic inflammatory disease (PID), which can cause infertility or chronic pelvic pain.	Antibiotics such as azithromycin. Treat partners, too.
Gonorrhea	Often asymptomatic; may cause burning during urination, vaginal discharge or bleeding	Can lead to PID, which can cause infertility or chronic pelvic pain.	Antibiotics such as ceftriaxone. Treat partners, too.
Syphilis	One sore may appear on genitals. Later symptoms include rash, muscle pain and hair loss.	Left untreated, it can lead to tumors on skin, liver or other organs, and cause blindness.	An injection of penicillin. Treat partners, too.
Trichomoniasis	Often asymptomatic; may cause vaginal discharge, odor and pain during urination and sex	Among pregnant women who have the STD, it can increase the risk of preterm delivery.	The oral antibiotic metronidazole
VIRAL			
Genital herpes	The first outbreak may cause lesions and flulike symptoms.	You or a partner can pass on the infection even if no sores are present, and you have it for life.	Antiviral drugs can ease pain and reduce outbreaks.
Hepatitis B and C	Often asymptomatic; both may cause nausea, fatigue, vomiting, stomach pain and jaundice.	Both cause liver inflammation and, in some cases, death. B (and often C) are lifelong conditions.	Prevent B with a vaccine; treat C with drugs.
HIV	Symptoms, which can take more than 10 years to appear, include weight loss, fatigue and fever.	HIV is a lifelong illness that can lead to AIDS (acquired immunodeficiency syndrome).	Antiviral medications can slow progression.
Human papillomavirus (HPV)	Warts may develop on genitals; sometimes the only sign of infection is an abnormal Pap.	Certain types of HPV can increase a woman's risk of developing cervical cancer.	A vaccine prevents it; topical cream or surgery treats it.

⏱ GOT 1 MINUTE?
Convince him to wear a condom

Some men will try any excuse to skip protection. Here's how to respond to their "I don't want to wear one" protests:

HE SAYS		YOU SAY
"I don't have one."	»	"I do." Keep a stash in your bedside table.
"If you loved me, you wouldn't ask me to wear one."	»	"If you love me, you'll wear it."
"But aren't you protected?"	»	"Against what? Pregnancy? It doesn't matter because tonight we're using a condom. But later on, we can both get tested for STDs. Sound good?"
"It will ruin the mood."	»	"I always use a condom, and the less worried I am about catching something, the easier it will be for me let loose in bed." Watch how fast he puts one on!

⏱ GOT 1 MINUTE?
Decide whether to come clean about your health

ONE IN FOUR American women will contract an STD in her lifetime. The big question: Should you tell your partner if you're one of them? Rather than mulling it over for weeks or even months, you can decide whether or not to disclose in less than 60 seconds. Here's how:

YOU SHOULD TELL IF it's incurable and/or communicable. Sit your partner down, preferably in a quiet place and before you've both stripped down to your skivvies, and tell him what you have, whether it's curable and how you can prevent transmission. He'll likely appreciate the honesty, and if not, better to find out early.

YOU DON'T HAVE TO TELL IF it's been treated and your doctor says you're cured or it's incommunicable. There's no need to share something that is ancient history and won't affect your partner.

⏱ GOT 5 MINUTES?
Request an STD test

Think your pelvic exam always includes an STD check? Not so fast. A Pap smear detects changes caused by infection, but it's not an STD test. In fact, the *American Journal of Public Health* reports that fewer than one third of doctors routinely screen for STDs. Discuss your history and the tests you should have with your ob/gyn.

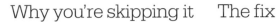

🕐 GOT 15 MINUTES?

Bust out of any dry spell

It's been a while since you've had sex. OK, truth be told, it's been so long that you've almost forgotten that, yes, you actually enjoy it. Here's how to address the reasons you're playing hooky from nooky—and strategies to help get you back into action.

Why you're skipping it

The fix

You've lost momentum. Every so often, you fall into a rut for no reason. Classic example: People who haven't had sex since their baby was born...and that baby now knows long division.

Blow the subject wide open. "Talking about it is the difference between being in a dry spell and being an ostrich with its head buried in the sand," says Sallie Foley, a sex therapist at the University of Michigan at Ann Arbor. "People worry that saying, 'We're not having sex' will cement it. But you're starting the process of connecting in a loving way."

You have no time. With eating and sleeping wedged between work and socializing, it's tough to squeeze in sex. "On the hierarchy of needs, sex isn't as crucial as sleep and food," Foley says.

Put it at the top of your to do list. Schedule sex the same as you would any other important meeting. "There's a myth of spontaneity," Foley explains. "When you make a reservation at a really nice restaurant, it doesn't take away from the pleasure of eating there." The same goes for sex: Planning it doesn't dampen the enjoyment factor.

You're distracted. Putting in long days at the office and being wired after hours aren't exactly conducive to a sex-friendly environment. BlackBerrys and cell phones are libido zappers!

Tune out the noise, turn off the computer and hop into bed earlier. If you and he regularly get sucked into television and wind up too tired to have sex, invest in TiVo—and swap the drama on the small screen for satisfaction in your bedroom. If you're zonked, turn in and try hitting it in the morning, instead of hitting the snooze button.

You're stretched too thin. Between working all day and being social with everyone, women may get disconnected from themselves—and deprived of rest, exercise and sex.

Reassign some chores. "Resentment at an uneven distribution of responsibilities tamps down desire," Foley explains. Have a frank talk and explain to your partner that he can help get you in the mood by vacuuming or sorting laundry. Or suggest that if he washed the floor (on his hands and knees), you would find that especially arousing.

You have no privacy. Your kids are omnipresent, and each year "they get more mobile and aware," says therapist Elana Katz of New York City. Sex is a no-go with little ears and eyes all around.

Barter child care with friends who are in the same boat. Or try asking Grandma to ferry Junior to his softball game, then stay home and have a toss of your own. Worried about being overheard when curious kiddies are around? Marvin Gaye played at an elevated volume can have an arousing—and remarkably soundproofing—effect.

⊕ GOT 10 MINUTES?
Analyze your racy dreams

Follow these steps to help decode last night's steamy imagery so you can enjoy sexier (real-life) sex tonight.

1 **JOT IT DOWN** Keep a notepad and pen by your bed to record details—setting, weather, objects, people, dialogue, feelings—while they're still fresh in your mind.

2 **BE LIKE SHERLOCK** For added insight, look up memorable images in a dream encyclopedia.

3 **TRUST YOUR INSTINCTS** There is more than one interpretation to a dream. If one doesn't feel right, read on until you find an explanation that hits a chord.

4 **NOTICE HOW YOU FEEL WHEN YOU AWAKEN** Had a hot dream about you and Johnny Depp and woke up grinning? Simply a satisfying dream. But if the star looked like your bitter ex and you woke up feeling sick, try to figure out what brought those feelings back to life.

5 **PHONE A FRIEND** Baffled? Run dreams by an old pal, who can help you recall events you've forgotten.

⊕ GOT 15 MINUTES?
Play NC-17 Pictionary

One surefire way to get sparks flying? A little creative use of your favorite board game. You and your partner can scribble down a list of terms or directives such as "Shower with me" or "Massage my feet" on cards, then take turns drawing them. Be sure to keep score so the victor can claim the grand prize: the opportunity to act out her favorite correctly guessed phrase.

⊕ GOT 8 MINUTES?
Stash an emergency intimacy kit

Every household should have the following good-sex necessities on hand, in case you—surprise!—unexpectedly find yourself stuck indoors with your sweetie with absolutely nothing to do.

☐ Condoms or your choice of birth control

☐ A bottle of red wine: Room temperature is fine.

☐ Batteries: They're not only for flashlights anymore.

☐ Candles: Use for mood lighting (or during a power outage!).

☐ Lacy, flirty undergarments: Need we say more?

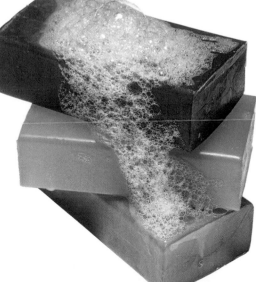

⏱ GOT 12 MINUTES? Figure out if your body is baby-ready

If you're yearning to be pregnant, don't let conception concerns keep you from fully delighting in sex. Take this quiz to get a quick snapshot of your pregnancy potential, then share the results with your ob/gyn, who can help you maximize your chances.

Which describes your menstrual cycle when you're not on the Pill?
a Like clockwork **3 points**
b Not the same each month, but I get a period every 24 to 35 days. **1 point**
c About as predictable as the stock market **–2 points**

Your score _____

How old are you?
a 35 or younger **3 points**
b Between 36 and 39 **1 point**
c 40 or older **–1 point**

Your score _____

Have you ever been pregnant?
a Yes, I'm already a mom. **2 points**
b Yes, but the pregnancy didn't go to term. **1 point**
c No **0 points**

Your score _____

Do you smoke?
a Yes, every day **–3 points**
b Occasionally/I've quit. **–1 point**
c No, and I never have. **2 points**

Your score _____

How much alcohol do you drink each week?
a 21 or more drinks **–2 points**
b 5 to 20 drinks **–1 point**
c Four or fewer drinks **1 point**

Your score _____

How much caffeine do you consume a day?
a At least five cups of coffee (or the equivalent in soda or tea, which have about a third of the caffeine) **–2 points**
b Three or four cups **–1 point**
c No more than two cups **1 point**

Your score _____

How often do you use artificial lubricants during sex, or do you use vaginal douches?
a Frequently **–2 points**
b Once in a while **–1 point**
c Rarely or never **1 point**

Your score _____

Have you ever had an STD?
a Yes. It was treated early. **0 points**
b Yes, and it wasn't treated until it was at a late stage. **–2 points**
c Maybe. I'm not sure. **–1 point**
d No. I'm screened regularly. **1 point**

Your score _____

Rate your stress level.
a I feel overwhelmed trying to juggle everything I have to do. **–2 points**
b I get stressed, but I exercise and practice relaxation techniques. **1 point**
c I hardly ever feel stressed at all. **0 points**

Your score _____

How often do you take a multivitamin with folic acid?
a Every day **1 point**
b When I remember **0 points**
c Never **–1 point**

Your score _____

How much vigorous exercise do you get each week?
a Seven or more hours **–1 point**
b Four to six hours **1 point**
c Three or fewer hours **0 points**

Your score _____

Do you think you may have an eating disorder?
a Yes **–3 points**
b In the past, but not now **0 points**
c No **1 point**

Your score _____

What's your body-mass index? (See page 254 to calculate your BMI.)
a 27 or higher **–2 points**
b 20 to 26 **2 points**
c Lower than 20 **–2 points**

Your score _____

What is your overall mood?
a Usually blue or anxious **–2 points**
b Some lows, but I'm OK. **0 points**
c Perfectly fine **1 point**

Your score _____

TOTAL SCORE: _____

What your score means

11 to 21 It looks as if your body and mind are primed for pregnancy. Enjoy the ride!

0 to 10 You might have a few issues to focus on. Some changes you may be able to tackle on your own—such as losing a few pounds or taking a multivitamin every day. Other concerns, such as having an erratic cycle, untreated depression or painful periods, may require your doctor's advice.

Less than 0 Consider putting the baby plans on hold for a while. You might have some habits, such as smoking, that could make it hard to conceive or could put a fetus at risk. See your ob/gyn for tips on preparing for pregnancy.

⏱ GOT 2 MINUTES?

Track your rhythm

Changes in your cervical fluid throughout the month can indicate when you're at your most fertile. What to look for if you want to conceive:

• After your period ends, your vagina and underwear will usually feel dry for several days. Your fertility is low.

• About a week later, you'll typically develop a sticky, gummy paste, which tends to be white or yellow. Still low.

• Secretions become creamy and lotionlike a few days later. Getting close.

• As you near ovulation, you'll produce a slippery, clear, egg white–like fluid. (Sperm love it because they swim right through.) Now is the time to go for it! Ovulation usually occurs on the final, or peak, day of slippery discharge.

• The egg lives for only about 24 hours once it's released, so it's best to have lots of sex the few days before ovulation. Sperm, on the other hand, can live for as long as four days waiting for their prize.

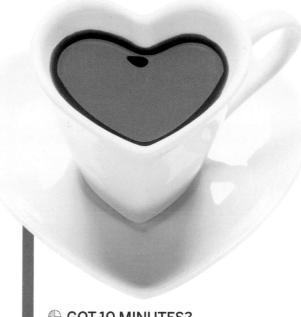

⏱ GOT 10 MINUTES?

Savor that java without worry

YOU DON'T HAVE to swear off your lattes if you're trying to conceive or are already pregnant. Only high doses of caffeine may make implantation difficult or increase the risk for miscarriage, says Carolyn Givens, M.D., co-medical director at the Pacific Fertility Center in San Francisco. So, go on. If you're jonesing for a jolt, have up to two cups of coffee (or its equivalent in soda or tea) a day. It's fine!

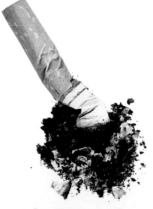

⏱ GOT 15 MINUTES?

Start thinking about quitting

Sure, you know that smoking cigarettes is dangerous for a developing fetus, but puffing can also make it more difficult for women to get pregnant in the first place. "Smoking is toxic to your eggs," Dr. Givens says. "If you smoke, you will lose your egg quality at a younger age." Do your best to break free of butts well before you attempt to conceive; your doctor can help you map out a step-by-step plan to kick the habit as well as advise you about which cessation aids aren't appropriate to continue using once you do get pregnant. For extra support online, visit QuitNet.com.

🕐 GOT 15 MINUTES (OR LESS)?

Set the scene for sex Candlelight? Bubble bath? Nice in theory, but not always realistic for that middle-of-the-week moment you're able to steal away with your partner. More doable: the following get-in-the-mood ideas, which will not only goose your libido but also help guarantee you'll make sex happen when you want it.

15 MIN · Stage a sexy scavenger hunt

First, squirrel away a half dozen suggestive items. Hide a lacy undergarment, a sensual snack, a sex toy or something that reminds him of a private naughty joke you share. Then write a starter note meant to lead him to the location of the first goody, and attach similar notes to hidden items. In addition to leading the seeker to the next item, the attached note might also provide explicit instruction for how you would like him to use the found object. Tell him when he's getting hot, and pretty soon you'll both be.

9 MIN · Get ready for your close-up

Stage a mini photo shoot at home. When you're playing a persona for your partner, you may find it easier to let loose and vamp. Next, enjoy the sexy images you took together, or if you're too shy, simply savor the shoot and then let him ooh and ahh over the pictures alone. Rest assured that with a digital camera, you can always erase the snapshots afterward. Oh, and be sure to remember to empty the trash folder.

1 MIN · Hire help

You'd be amazed how a babysitter or house-keeper can revitalize your sex life. If you get some help around the house to lighten your mental load, you can make sex more of a priority. Do a quick calculation: How many extra minutes could you bank for a booty call if you didn't have to spend Saturday afternoon vacuuming every room, dusting every side table and mopping every floor? And how many would you have if you sent your kids to the playground with a sitter? Pick up the phone and make the call.

15 MIN · Read the signs

Here's a radical thought: You might be in the mood more often than you realize. Research indicates that many women don't recognize the bodily signs of sexual arousal—clitoral swelling and lubrication, for instance—while the symptoms are occurring. "Women who are more sexually active and report more sexual pleasure in their relationships are much more aware of these physical responses," explains psychologist

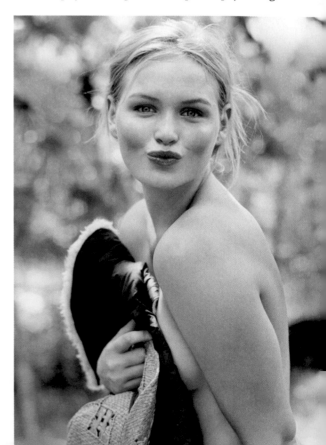

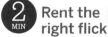

and sex therapist Robert Hatfield, Ph.D., spokesman for the Society of Scientific Study of Sexuality in Allentown, Pennsylvania. If you get to know your body's indications that you're sex-ready, your mood will follow much more often. Put aside 15 minutes to read a sexy book or watch a sexy video (preferably in the nude). Whenever you come across something titillating, wait a few moments to give your body a chance to respond. "You may be pleasantly surprised to discover sensations you'd previously been unaware of," Hatfield adds. With repeated practice, you'll learn to recognize your sexual responses even when you're not focused on them. Then you can—and we hope will—feel moved to act on them.

1 MIN Beat the sex slump

You might not imagine there's a connection between what you do all day and the sex you have at night, but research suggests there is: Nerve signals to the pelvic area travel best down a straight spine, so an upright posture "enhances the muscles and sensory function around the vagina," says the Berman Center's Laura Berman. Slouch regularly, and your organs could also press on and weaken critical pelvic-floor muscles. To improve your sex life, focus on making your body the shape of an exclamation point rather than a question mark.

15 MIN Take to the tub as a twosome

The secret to making bath time fun is not a rubber ducky; it's ice cubes. Take turns tracing patterns on each other's skin. The contrast between hot and cold can intensify physical sensations, possibly heightening arousal, says Linda Mona, Ph.D., a clinical psychologist in Los Angeles. Rub-a-dub-dub!

3 MIN Say, "Kudos to me!"

"Good sex comes from feeling positive about your identity as a whole," say sex therapist Sallie Foley. Before you hit the sheets, write down one accomplishment you're proud of and why you rocked at it. Maybe you ran 5 miles, helped out a friend who was feeling overwhelmed or polished off a big project at work. Bask in the glow of achievement and that confidence will spill over into the bedroom.

2 MIN Rent the right flick

At the video store, skip the new releases and head straight for the romantic comedies or dramas. A study in the journal *Hormones and Behavior* found that watching a romantic movie can raise progesterone levels 10 percent, which make you more touchy-feely. A good horror film might also encourage serious cuddling, according to research from Roanoke College in Salem, Virginia, which noted that couples who watched slasher movies together ended up in smooch sessions more often than those who attended a Mozart concert. So dim the lights, silence your cell phone, press play and shhh...absolutely no talking!

5 MIN Be a basket case

Place a basket or bowl outside your bedroom with a pad and pen inside and jot down things likely to invade your thoughts during sex—chores to do, petty beefs with your beefcake—items that have nothing to do with how much you love each other. You can leave your worries at the door. Address what's in the basket later, and focus on the good stuff now.

2 MIN Hot sync your hearts

Most women don't walk around aroused; instead, they become more amorous when reminded of how much they love their partner. To speed up the process, try soul gazing, a goofy but blissfully nonverbal way to get reacquainted after time apart: Close your eyes, hold hands and breathe together for 30 seconds, then switch to inhaling when he exhales. Imagine you're receiving love through his palms and sending him love through yours. You'll both feel more present. And don't worry, it's OK to giggle!

3 MIN Take a pledge

Promise that you'll do something simple to express yourself emotionally to your partner every day, such as squeezing his hand when you talk to him. Make it a habit and you'll ratchet up your connection.

1 MIN Kiss off a bad day

Create a new rule to give your sweetie a long, intense kiss when you both get home from work, no matter how dismal your day was. Hot hellos help you remember you're with someone you love and that the rest of the world is unimportant when you're locked in each other's embrace. Besides, it gives you something sexy to look forward to during your mundane commute. (Just do not miss your exit or train stop!)

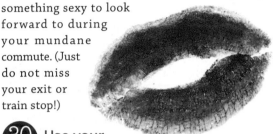

30 SEC Use your imagination

Thinking sultry thoughts can quickly ignite your sexual self-awareness. Instead of making a mental to do list while standing in line at the bank or grocery store, try envisioning a two-minute scenario with the hot customer in front of you. "Fantasy is a good way to keep sexuality alive, as long as you feel positive about it, not guilty," says John Bancroft, M.D., director of the Kinsey Institute for Research in Sex, Gender and Reproduction at Indiana University in Bloomington. Remember, it's a daydream to ponder, not a plan of action to pounce on.

15 MIN Reach out and touch

Undress and blindfold your guy, then give him a full-body massage. "The blindfold allows you to forget about your body-image hang-ups, but it's also sexy and mysterious," says Sheila Kelley, of Los Angeles, creator of S Factor, a pole-dancing workout. Let the massage lead to something more. "With no self-consciousness, you move out of instinct. The sex will knock your socks off."

10 MIN Phone it in

After spending some alone time in separate rooms reading or relaxing, send your mate a suggestive text message. Enjoying some sexually charged phone chatter may come a little easier when you're not face-to-face. "People often feel inhibited about conveying what they like and what they don't like sexually, and the phone can help you get over that discomfort," says Linda Mona, a psychologist in Los Angeles. For starters, try something like "4play is gr8" or "TDTM" (translation: Talk dirty to me).

3 MIN Do a sex-enhancing workout

Done regularly, Kegel exercises—completed by tensing and releasing the pelvic muscles as though you are trying to hold back urine flow—can heighten your enjoyment of intercourse. Lie on your back with knees bent, feet flat on the floor. Contract the pelvic muscles and hold for 10 seconds; release. Then do five quick contractions. Repeat the entire sequence for 3 minutes, working up to 10 minutes a day (broken into three separate sessions if you like).

5 MIN Hit replay

Mentally relive your favorite sexual memory. What do you see? Feel? Hear? Taste? Smell? The point is to visualize what turns you on—and often. "By the time you see your lover, you'll be so excited from all the intimate thoughts you've had," says Barbara Bartlik, M.D., professor of psychiatry at Weill Cornell Medical College in New York City. Whisper them in his ear, and watch his excitement level spike, too.

1 MIN Get mute-ual satisfaction

Sometimes, closing down one sense can heighten the others. Tonight, don't say a word to your partner during lovemaking. Eliminating any verbal communication forces you to read each other's body language. And focusing so intently on the act can make you feel more connected with each other.

2 MIN Swap stories

When you're in your partner's arms, but your mind is still at the office, ask him to listen to you without offering any feedback for five minutes, says Patricia Taylor, Ph.D., a sex counselor in Las Vegas. Talk about whatever is on your mind, then give him five minutes to share. "When you listen to each other without judgment, you feel valued and heard," she says. And once you've made that crucial emotional link to each other, your body will be ready to follow.

YOUR SEX TO-DON'T LIST

» Don't wear sweats to bed every night. Even if you're not in the mood, cuddling in the buff can ignite a spark.

» Don't watch late-night TV. The earlier you climb into bed, the more likely you'll have some energy for sex.

» Don't shoulder all the chores yourself. Ask your honey to pitch in around the house so you'll have more time to focus on him—in bed and out.

» Don't be afraid to experiment with new positions. Variety is one key to keeping passion in your sex life alive, so be brave about trying different ways.

» Don't be shy about scheduling sex. Penciling it in helps ensure it happens.

» Don't stay mum about your needs. Show and tell your partner exactly what you want in bed. It will help keep both of you more satisfied.

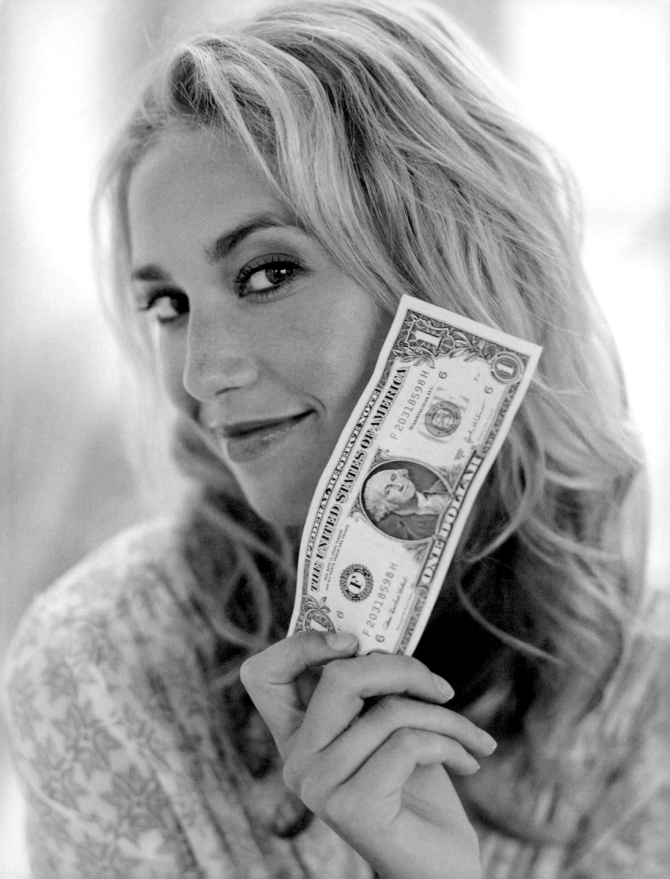

money maneuvers

CHAPTER
8

You can have all the finer things in life (and a decent cushion to spare) if you learn to manage your green judiciously. The next 18 pages will put an end to money stress, whatever your age or stage. These ingenious tips are designed to help you spend smartly, save painlessly—no scrimping or forgoing fun!—and invest your dough wisely so you can live a richer life today and in the years ahead.

The only 10 things you need to know about managing your money efficiently

When you need a fiver to buy a cappuccino, when a decent pair of jeans costs a Benjamin, when a starter house sets you back hundreds of thousands of dollars, you know it's time to be supersmart about your finances. Streamline spending and maximize savings with these money musts and you'll be living large in no time.

1 Know thy financial self

Before you plot your way to riches, you need a clear understanding of your current financial status, and that means calculating your net worth. (Use the worksheet on page 190 to find your number.) On average, a healthy net worth—your assets, including real estate, minus your debt—should equal your age times 10 percent of your pretax income. For example, a 25-year-old making $32,000 annually can consider herself in good financial shape if she's worth $80,000.

2 Track your spending

To take control of your money, learn exactly where it goes. For two weeks, log how you spend every nickel, whether for pedicures or parking meters. Divide the expenses into categories, such as bills, beauty and transportation. Then multiply each weekly spending category by 52, and don't faint. You're looking for the "insignificant" purchases that rack up thousands. (That $150 you drop every weekend on brunch, drinks, dinner, movies and maybe a teensy bit of shopping? It equals $7,800 a year.)

3 Start an SOS fund

Give yourself a cushion. If you're ever laid off and depend on plastic, it could take years to recover. Aim to have three months of living expenses on reserve. Put what you can (shoot for 10 percent of your total paycheck each month) into a savings account that earns at least 4 percent interest. Add to the kitty by throwing singles in a tin and depositing them once it's full. Your sense of security will grow, too.

4 Banish bad debt

"Good" debt, such as a mortgage or student loan, increases long-term earning power. Credit card debt puts you in a hole. Get out of it starting here.
- **Lay off the cards.** Put them in a bowl of water and shove the whole thing in your freezer.
- **Negotiate lower rates.** Often, all it takes is asking. Or threaten to switch to a low-interest card. (Would you pay 20 percent more for everything? That's what you do carrying a balance on a high-interest card.)
- **Up your outlay.** Exceed your required minimum, and you'll reduce the principal, not merely cover interest.

5 Pump up your paycheck

By not asking for a higher salary at work, you may cheat yourself out of hundreds of thousands of dollars in the long run. Hard to believe? If, at age 22, you get an offer for $25K and negotiate it to $30K, then annually put the difference into an account earning 3 percent interest a year, you'll accrue $568,834 by age 60 (assuming you receive an annual raise of 3 percent—a conservative estimate—and increase your savings accordingly). To be an ace negotiator, give three reasons you're worth more than the next gal. If your employer won't budge, ask to tie a bonus to a specific project. Or interview elsewhere; even if you ultimately don't switch jobs, you can use a competing offer to leverage a raise.

6 Build a retirement nest egg

To avoid subsisting on early bird specials later, augment your SOS fund by saving another 12 percent of your income every year until you retire, says Charles Farrell, a financial consultant in Medina, Ohio. A 401(k) is the best place to put it. If your employer doesn't offer one, contribute the annual maximum to an individual retirement account and invest it in a mutual fund geared for retirement. If you're in debt, have the bank transfer $50 a week into savings. In six months, you'll have enough to open a brokerage account. Invest it, and let your money work for you.

7 Lower your expenses

Even among dual-earning families, bankruptcies are too common, in part because couples spend both paychecks, making themselves vulnerable if one income disappears. If you're part of a two-income household, allocate half of your total income to mortgage, taxes, utilities, gas, food and insurance, 12 percent to retirement, 10 percent to rainy-day savings and the rest to clothes, vacations and other luxuries. If you're the sole breadwinner, set up automatic transfers at your bank. If you put $25 per biweekly paycheck into an account earning 4.6 percent interest, in five years, you'll have earned $3,316 to put toward a down payment or into your SOS fund.

8 Double your dollar confidence

Rather than stressing about the perfect financial life, do what you can today. Can't save $10,000? Save $1,000. Don't have time to plow through the minutiae of your retirement plan? Sign up for it now, and put your money in a target-date fund, which automatically allocates money based on when you plan to retire. You don't need to understand the intricacies of price-earnings ratios to have the financial life you want. You're fully capable of getting a grip on your dollars—just do it one step at a time.

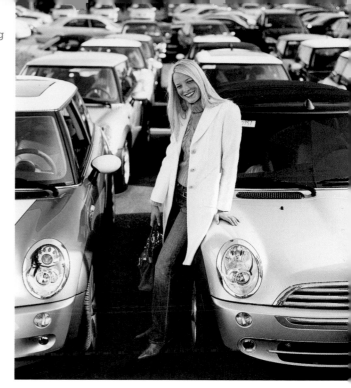

9 Envision your future

Once you have your financial present in order, write down short- and long-term goals. Do you want to launch your own business? Retire in Tuscany? Then figure out a time frame and a price tag and plot what you need to do to achieve your dream. Use an online calculator to crunch numbers. Or talk to a financial planner; see page 195 for help finding one.

10 Keep it in perspective

Remember, money really doesn't buy happiness. In one study, researchers at Northwestern University in Evanston, Illinois, found that people who won up to a million bucks in the lottery not only were no happier a year after collecting their jackpot than nonwinners, but they also took less pleasure in daily activities. Take a moment or two to list what you value most. Chances are, your family, friends and health will rank higher than an Hermès bag. Then think about how to use your money to help nurture your values and pursue life goals. Take a weekend getaway with friends so you can build memories together. Join a gym so you feel healthier and more energized. Give to your favorite charity. Let your spending reflect your beliefs, and your life—not to mention your wallet—will feel a whole lot fuller.

⏱ GOT 10 MINUTES?
Protect your identity

THE FEDERAL TRADE commission logged 246,035 complaints of credit-damanging identity theft in 2006—and that's only the cases that were reported to authorities. Take one simple step to avoid being a victim of this crime: Buy a shredder so you can slice any financial paperwork before throwing it out. Find more ways you can protect yourself below.

● Never send your complete Social Security number or credit card number over e-mail or via an insecure website. (Look for the padlock symbol to be sure.)
● Once a year, order your credit report free from Annual CreditReport.com, a central credit report service that compiles reports from the three agencies that maintain them (Equifax, Experian and TransUnion). Check the reports to be sure you are familiar with any credit accounts or debts recorded there.
● If someone does abuse your credit card, notify the credit card company immediately and place a fraud alert on your credit report. An initial alert lasts 90 days, but if you've been the victim of identity theft, you can now put a seven-year notice in your file.

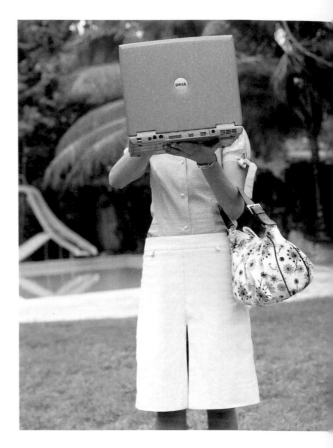

⏱ GOT 7 MINUTES?
Compute your net worth Are you moving in the right direction, moneywise? Crunch these numbers at least once a year to get an instant snapshot of how much progress you've made.

$ _____	**Cash**	Add all bank accounts, stocks, bonds, mutual funds, retirement savings and life insurance policies with cash value.
+ _____	**Property**	Add the current value of your home, other real estate and your car. (Visit Edmunds.com for a quote on the last one.)
+ _____	**Personal belongings**	Add the value of jewelry, antiques, art, collections and other big-ticket items you could sell.
− _____	**Debt**	Subtract the sum of the mortgage on your home, credit card debt, student and car loans and other money you owe.
$ _____	**TOTAL**	This is your net worth. For tips on how to increase it, visit www.360financialliteracy.org/women.

🕑 GOT 2 MINUTES?

Learn how to free yourself from debt

Debt can be smart if you're borrowing at low, tax-favored rates to buy a house. But if you're heavily in debt on your credit cards, this is your recovery strategy:

1 **STOP USING YOUR CREDIT CARDS** Cut them up if you have to, but cut yourself off.

2 **KNOW WHAT YOU'RE FACING** Make a chart listing the amounts, interest rates, minimum payments due and customer service phone numbers for each card.

3 **GET A BETTER RATE** Interest matters. If you have a $10,000 balance on a card that charges 15 percent, you're losing $1,500 a year in interest alone. Call each of your card companies and ask for a lower rate. If they won't budge, transfer your balance to a new card with the lowest rate offered (zero, if possible). Go to CardWeb .com to research rates.

4 **PAY MORE** Identify the card with the highest rate, and figure out how much you can spare each month beyond the minimum to pay it down. Paying off $10,000 at $300 a month instead of $200 can cut your debt repayment by nearly three years. See BankRate.com to run the numbers.

🕑 GOT 30 SECONDS?

Check if you're covered

You have car and health insurance, but what about homeowners/renters, life and disability insurance? Visit Insure.com for quotes on a policy.

🕑 GOT 5 MINUTES?

Slash a bill

Shop better and you'll save a few bucks, but lower your regular household bills and you'll save a few bucks a month. A smart place to get started: LowerMyBills.com, which helps consumers find the best deals on cell phones, Internet access, mortgages and more.

🕑 GOT 15 MINUTES?

Write a will

No one wants to think about making a will, and it's easy to put it off until you have a million bucks. But should you die unexpectedly without a will, the state will write one for you— and decide, on your behalf, who gets your assets and who takes care of pets or even your kids, if you have them. You don't need a lawyer to draft a basic will, which should suffice if you're younger than 40 and won't be subject to estate taxes. Go for software, such as Quicken's WillMaker Plus.

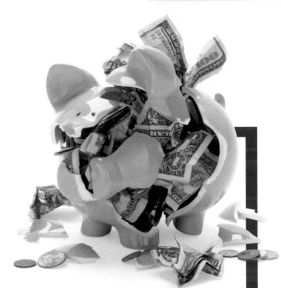

🕐 GOT 13 MINUTES?
Sign up for your retirement plan

If your employer offers you a 401(k) or 403(b) retirement plan, sign up for it right now. You may be decades away from retirement or unable to put away the recommended 12 percent; that's OK. "If you don't have any money in a retirement plan, start by depositing 1 percent of each paycheck, then increase it to 2 percent, then 3 percent and so on. You can do small things that start to change your ways," says Dee Lee, a certified financial planner in Harvard, Massachusetts. By doing so, you'll get a triple whammy: First, you'll have the money you'll need to live well in retirement. Second, you'll reap a nice tax break. And third, many companies offer a match so if you put a certain amount toward retirement, your employer will do the same. Think of it this way: By not contributing, you could be throwing away thousands of dollars in free money!

🕐 GOT 5 MINUTES?
Put savings on autopilot

WHEN IT COMES to finances, one of the simplest and most effective things you can do is schedule a monthly automatic deposit from your paycheck or checking account into a savings account or mutual fund. Ask your payroll department at work to arrange automatic increases in your savings when your income grows. A 2004 study conducted by behavioral finance professors from leading business schools found that people who agreed up front to increase the percentage of income they set aside for retirement each time they got a raise (and had to opt out to undo that decision) increased their savings rate from 3.5 percent to 11.6 percent in a mere two years and four months.

🕐 GOT 15 MINUTES?
Collect for your kids' college

If you have kids, you probably know private college averages upwards of $30,000 a year. Set up a 529 savings plan—which allows you to save tax-free for kids' college years—while your tots are still in diapers. There's a slew of plans out there; start your search by looking at your home state's plan, because many states offer state tax benefits in addition to the federal ones.

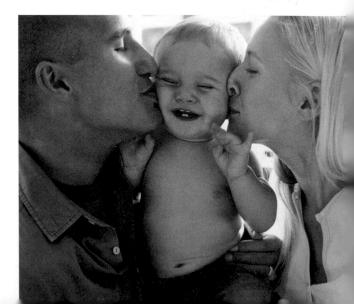

⊕ GOT 6 MINUTES?

Learn where to stash your cash
Stocks can be great for long-term savings, but they are also often volatile. Bonds are solid but slow-growing. The lowdown on what kinds of savings should go where:

	PROS	CONS	RETURNS	BEST FOR
Savings accounts and money market funds	Safety	Low returns	Savings earn from 0.5 percent to 5 percent for online accounts. Money markets average 4 percent.	Immediate needs (such as your summer vacation) and emergency funds
Stocks and stock funds	Higher returns	Volatility	Historically 10 percent	Retirement, longer-term savings
Bonds and bond funds	Relative safety, minimal volatility	Relatively low returns	Historically 5 percent	Lowering the risk of your overall portfolio

⊕ GOT 8 MINUTES?
Mesh your money personalities

If you're a saver and your spouse is a spender, try creating separate lists of your short- and long-term financial goals, then compare notes. If you're not in sync, focus on the top two items for each of you and work together. It might be easier for you to commit to a pricey vacation, for example, if he agrees that you'll both save for it for at least six months.

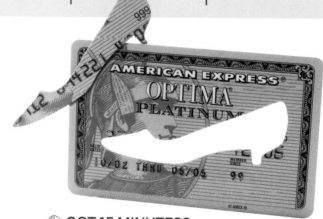

⊕ GOT 15 MINUTES?
Go on a spending diet

Scan six months of credit card and bank statements to help you suss out spending spikes. Did your American Express bill skyrocket during times of stress? If so, consider calming your emotions in ways that don't involve money, such as spending time with close friends. To forestall your worst impulse spending, leave your wallet (or at least your credit cards) locked in your desk when you window-shop at lunch.

🕐 GOT 10 MINUTES? Master the basics of retirement funds

Selecting investments for your 401(k) can feel overwhelming. "But researching options can mean the difference between retiring on the beach and scrounging for rent," says personal finance expert Laura Rowley of Maplewood, New Jersey.

Know the formula

To gauge how much you should be putting into stock-based mutual funds, which are riskier but generate more interest, versus bond funds, which are more stable but usually less profitable, subtract your age from 100; then put that percentage of your contribution in stocks, the rest in bonds. (If you're 30, that means you'll be investing 70 percent in stocks, 30 percent in bonds.)

Mix it up

Next, put 70 percent of your stock allocation in a large-cap fund (i.e., one investing in big companies), 20 percent in mid-cap and 10 percent in small-cap. Also, select a mixture of growth, value and blended funds. Growth funds carry risk but may earn more, value funds are conservative and blends fall in the middle. "There's no right or wrong," Rowley says. "It's about your appetite for risk."

Run a background check

Go to Morningstar.com and use the data interpreter to rate your fund. Avoid funds ranked two stars or less. Look for a below-average expense ratio (to reduce fees) and a manager who's been with the fund for at least five years. From those, look under Trailing Returns for funds that match or beat the stated benchmark, such as the S&P 500, over five years. Then watch your nest egg grow.

🕐 GOT 3 MINUTES?
Scout out hidden fees

THE CHARGES ATTACHED to some mutual funds can really eat into your holdings. Fees are expressed as a percent of assets known as expense ratios. If a fund's expense ratio (found in its prospectus) is 1.5 percent, that means it charges $15 a year for every $1,000 invested. If you invest $1,000 and get a return of 8 percent in a year, you've made $80 gross. But then you pay nearly 20 percent of your gain in fees. And if the fund goes down, you still pay those fees. Ouch. (Most funds that are sold by brokers also charge a sales fee that's paid either when you buy or when you sell.) You can buy an index fund for rock-bottom fees of only 0.19 percent or any number of standout actively managed funds for between 0.5 percent and 1 percent.

🕐 GOT 1 MINUTE?
See how your green can grow

Save early and you can easily become a millionaire, all thanks to the power of compounding. New gains are based not only on your original investment, but also on any interest you have already earned. But the longer you wait, the harder it is to amass a fortune. Here's how much you'll need to save each month in a retirement account to become a millionaire by 65, assuming an annualized 9 percent return:

Make your first million

YOUR AGE	MONTHLY SAVINGS
25	$214
35	$547
45	$1,500

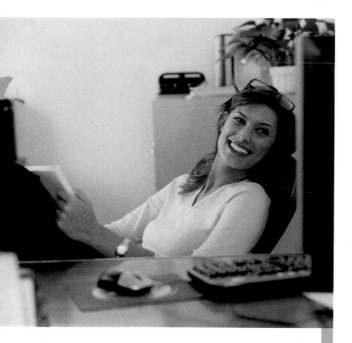

⏱ GOT 15 MINUTES?
Consider consulting a financial expert

MAYBE YOU FEEL perfectly comfortable buying stocks or funds on your own. But if you crave more hand-holding, here are some tips for hiring a financial advisor.

● **Start with a referral** from a friend or family member. If no promising names turn up through personal connections, check in with the National Association of Personal Financial Advisors at NAPFA.org.

● **Do a little due diligence.** You can check out any stockbroker's background for free at BrokerCheck .NASD.com; if your advisor is not a broker, scope out her background, disciplinary record, fees and investment strategies for free at AdviserInfo.SEC.gov.

● **Interview your prospective advisor.** Ask about her background and credentials and whether she works with clients in your stage of life and with your portfolio size. You'll also need someone with whom you feel comfortable talking and who will listen to you. Also consider how your advisor is being paid. A fee-only advisor (who is paid only by clients, sometimes based on a percentage of assets) is generally far preferable to a commission-based broker (who might be tempted to push products just to earn a buck).

⏱ GOT 4 MINUTES?
Pick up the lingo

Don't speak Wall Street? Get started with the list below, then visit InvestorWords.com and subscribe to its "Financial Term of the Day" via e-mail.

ACTIVELY MANAGED A fund for which a manager chooses stocks, versus computer models. Managers often do not outperform the market, so do your homework before buying.

EDGAR Available at SEC.gov, this free database compiles corporate information.

MARKET CAP A measure of a company's size. A large-cap company has a capitalization of more than $10 billion and tends to carry less risk.

MARKET INDEX A group of representative stocks (like the 30 stocks on the Dow Jones Industrial Average) used to gauge the health of the market.

NO-LOAD A fund on which your broker does not earn a commission, saving you fees.

PROSPECTUS Everything about a mutual fund can be found in this document: goals, strategies, risks, fees and past performance. Request one before investing, and get advice on how to read it at SEC.gov.

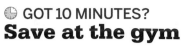

🕐 GOT 9 MINUTES?
Cut Rx costs

NEARLY ONE IN four Americans says that she or a family member has cut pills in half or failed to fill a prescription in the past year because of the expense, according to a survey by *USA Today*, the Harvard School of Public Health in Boston and the Kaiser Family Foundation in Menlo Park, California. Follow our prescription for lower drug costs.

In the doctor's office Ask your M.D. about cheaper drug options. A generic or older, tried-and-true medication may work just as well as a pricier brand, so guide the conversation to dollars and cents the next time your physician whips out her pad and pen.

When you purchase If you fill prescriptions online, cut the price of your medication by visiting PharmacyChecker .com, a site that scours the Internet for the best deals on brand-name drugs. (Order only from a reputable site that requires your doctor's Rx.) Rather not buy online? Ask your pharmacist to match the price you spotted on the Web—some will negotiate to keep your business.

🕐 GOT 10 MINUTES?
Save at the gym

● Ask your friends and colleagues how much they're paying for their gym membership. You will quickly find out that two members of the same club may pay vastly different prices. Before you sign up, demand a deal as good as your luckier pal's. Industry insiders say gyms will often match the fee, but not unless you ask.

● Another tactic: Wait until the 30th of the month. Sales reps typically have monthly goals, so as they try to sign you up on the spot, they'll often sweeten the deal with free introductory periods, lower initiation fees or free personal training sessions.

● There's no need to sweat huge monthly trainer's fees. "It takes only three meetings for a trainer to design a program, which you can then do on your own," says Juan Carlos Santana, director of the Institute of Human Performance in Boca Raton, Florida. But be sure to check in several times a year to tweak your regimen.

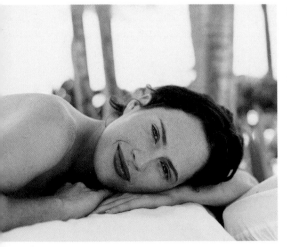

🕐 GOT 6 MINUTES?
Enjoy a free massage

If you're injured or ill, let your insurer pay for a rubdown. With a scrip from your doctor, major health insurers may pay for medically required massages. Just ask: "Policies cover more than they publicize, but you won't get certain benefits unless you request them," says Kevin Flynn, president of Healthcare Advocates in Philadelphia. Weight issues? Nutritional counseling and gym memberships can be reimbursable, too, if you simply assert yourself.

⏱ GOT 4 MINUTES? Shrink your shrink bills and dental costs

Regular visits to a specialist can eat into your medical budget. Consider these cash-conserving alternatives if you often seek help from a therapist or dentist.

BOOK CHEAPER COUCH TIME Instead of paying through the nose (and often out of pocket) for therapy, get it via a psychology or psychiatry graduate-degree training program, offered at most large universities. You'll receive the undivided attention of a professionally supervised therapist completing her education, says SELF's mental-health expert, Catherine Birndorf, M.D. Bring your pay stub to your appointment; fees are often based on a sliding scale (as opposed to the triple-digit hourly rates many psychotherapists charge).

OPEN WIDE FOR DISCOUNT DENTAL WORK Similarly, you can take a bite out of dental expenses by searching for a local dental school at ADA.org. Students (monitored by faculty) do almost everything, from general cleanings to fixing a chipped tooth. You'll save 50 to 60 percent. Appointments are often in the early morning or evening and can last twice as long as at a dentist's office. (Professors must review students' work.) But the time you invest does dull the pain of paying for that root canal in full.

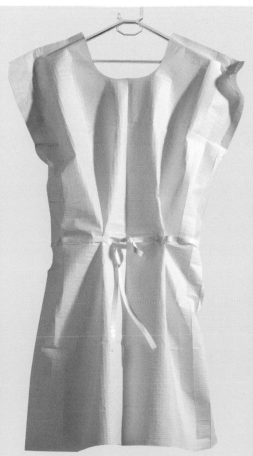

⏱ GOT 2 MINUTES?
Avoid medical debt
Millions of middle-class Americans have been recently bankrupted by health problems. Protect yourself before you reach the hospital door.

NEVER GO UNINSURED If you can't afford the best policy, get one with a very high deductible that covers catastrophic illnesses or accidents. Visit Insure.com to compare policies.

KNOW WHAT'S COVERED Ask your insurer if it imposes any caps on what it will pay, either annually or over your lifetime, and whether certain drugs or treatments aren't covered. You can't fill the gaps in your plan unless you know what they are.

INVESTIGATE YOUR OPTIONS If you enter the hospital and know you may have trouble covering your bills, ask immediately to speak with an in-house financial counselor to learn what your insurance covers and whether you qualify for any price breaks or aid. Don't be embarrassed, and don't hesitate to make a ruckus if you aren't getting the help you need.

FIND AN ADVOCATE Consult the resources on debt at ConsumerLaw.org. Locate a lawyer or nonprofit counselor through the local bar association, Legal Services office or the National Association of Consumer Advocates at NACA.net.

⏱ GOT 15 MINUTES (OR LESS)?

Discover secret ways to save There are so many tricks to nab a deal—if you know how to navigate the retail jungle. Allow us to provide a map.

① MIN Seal the deal

If you're looking to negotiate a purchase price, swap that smile for a surly grimace. Apparently, heated hagglers get better prices than chipper types, reports the *Journal of Personality and Social Psychology.* The caveat: The less-than-affable approach may work only with strangers, so try it when hunting flea market bargains, not when buying a friend's car.

② MIN Shop by yourself

The mere presence of fellow shoppers can sway us to shell out for a fancy label, possibly because we don't want to be seen as cheap, a study in the *Journal of Consumer Research* reveals. Avoid overspending by considering your purchase solo before buying.

⑤ MIN Take a preshopping breather

If you're feeling cranky, go for a soothing walk before you hit the mall. Angry people may be less apt to compare prices, especially on big-ticket items, than folks who are feeling sad or neutral, researchers at the University of Pittsburgh say.

③⓪ SEC Buy full-price, guilt-free

Gotta have it? Grab it! Many stores, including J.Crew, Saks and Barneys, will refund the difference if your duds go on sale within a week (or even later). Ask about the price-adjustment policy, and keep the receipt.

② MIN Click to be chic

eBay is a virtual fashion mecca, thanks in part to New Yorkers who sell the clothes they've bought at designer sample sales. Ask the site to e-mail you whenever your favorite label goes on the auction block, and consult advice on the site on how to avoid scams and make sure you've nabbed an authentic item.

⑮ MIN Grab sneaks for a song

Get your kicks in June, when shops stock next season's styles. "Ask the store when the latest shoes come out, then go a week later and buy the old model," says Cynthia Krieger, manager of See Jane Run Sports in San Francisco. "Shoe styles change gradually, so the only difference you're likely to notice is the price."

② MIN Trade in your gifts

If you haven't spent that last holiday gift card, send it to SwapAGift.com to cash it in for up to 75 percent of its value, depending on the store. Or check out CertificateSwap.com, a site that sells unused gift certificates in exchange for cash—or lets you transform one gift card into another. Turn your The Children's Place credit into one from Anthropologie and get what *you* really want.

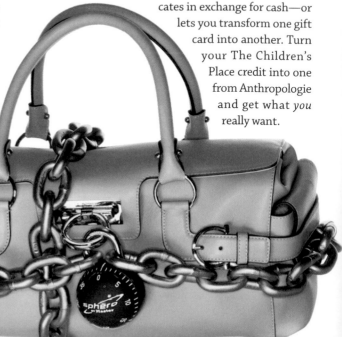

5 MIN Search for online freebies

Shopping in stores may be fun, but it's often a lot cheaper online. Go to CurrentCodes.com to find discount codes you can use at checkout for the latest deals. Or you can use PriceGrabber.com to find the cheapest price on whatever you're looking for.

7 MIN Let retailers reimburse you

Credit cards aren't the only way to get cash back; many retailers offer their own version of discount cards and cash-back offers. Get a Barnes & Noble card for $25 and get up to 40 percent off list price on hardcover best sellers. Join Staples for free and get 10 percent off ink, paper and various other items; then use the store's online rebate center to claim manufacturer rebates. Order toiletries from Drugstore.com and get cash back on your next order. Whatever your favorite retailers are, it's likely they have a rewards program. And you won't need to be a coupon fanatic to make it work for you.

5 MIN Customize your clothing

If you spot a Missoni sweater at a Kmart price, buy it, even if it's a tad too small, and then head to your dry cleaner. He may be able to stretch wool (including cashmere) and acrylic at least one and a half sizes through a process called knit blocking, says Chuck Horst, general manager of Margaret's Cleaners in La Jolla, California. For the cost of a cleaning, he'll steam and stretch the top until it fits like a dream.

4 MIN Hire a personal shopper

You don't need to troll Rodeo Drive to enjoy posh treatment, so why sift through racks when you can find someone to do it for you? Many major department stores offer free personal shopping services, regardless of the amount you spend. A cute new bikini for your vacay in Puerto Vallarta? ¡Sí, señorita!

13 MIN Maintain a perfect 10

Keep nails immaculate by booking cheapie polish changes—half the price of a full-scale mani or pedi. And BYOP: Purchase your own professional-grade polish and ask the manicurist to use your bottle, so you know you're getting fresh, top-quality polish

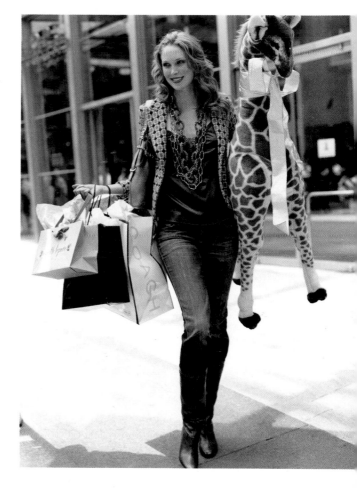

that won't chip as quickly. Plus, once you have your favorite shade at home for quick touch-ups, you won't have to return to the salon as often.

3 MIN Pay drugstore prices and get designer-worthy results

Splurge on good brushes, and you'll end up with makeup that looks luxe, even using drugstore brands, says makeup artist Rebecca Restrepo of New York City: "They help products go on evenly." Like many cosmetics cognoscenti, she loves the Shu Uemura line.

1 MIN Create a posh-looking pout

Make cheap lipstick seem custom-blended with this tip: When torn between hues, pick the darker. "You can fade it with gloss," says Nick Barose, a makeup artist in New York City.

⏱ GOT 15 MINUTES? Go exploring online

Seventy-nine million Americans make travel plans using the Internet each year, according to a report by the Travel Industry Association in Washington, D.C. To chart your next adventure, hit one of SELF's favorite websites, each with a different approach to help you find what you need. The trick to getting a deal: Do your research, and when you find a trip at the right price, don't bookmark it—buy it.

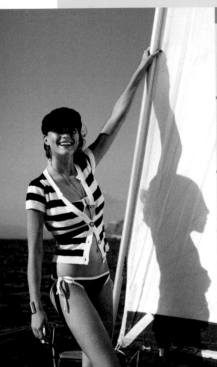

WEBSITE	GREAT FOR	WHAT IT DOES
Cheap Accommodation .com	Comparison shoppers looking for the best hotel rates	Reveals how amenities and prices stack up (e.g., three-star hotel versus villa versus bed-and-breakfast)
TripAdvisor.com	Travelers in search of unbiased reviews	Provides uncensored, tell-all critiques, insider tips and unairbrushed photographs from folks who've been there
Groople.com	Pals planning a journey together	Allows you to book group trips at group rates but lets each person pay individually
LastMinute.com	Last-minute vacationers	Lists grab-and-go deals for jetting off on a getaway up to three hours prior to takeoff
FareCompare .com	Flyers anxious about overpaying	Tracks airfares between 75 domestic destinations and predicts whether the price will rise or fall in the next week

⏱ GOT 15 MINUTES?
See Europe for a song

Low-cost airlines have revolutionized travel within Europe, offering fares as low as a few bucks from smaller airports in major cities such as London, Dublin or Amsterdam. Investigate routes and fares at RyanAir.com, EasyJet.com, Flybe .com or WizzAir.com. Book a cheap connecting flight, or jet around the continent for peanuts.

⏱ GOT 5 MINUTES?
Drive a luxury rental car

Weekend wheels rent for less in May, when car companies stock up, and in September, before they sell the fleets. Translation: "You can nab a deal while there's excess inventory," says Barbara Messing, travel expert for Hotwire.com.

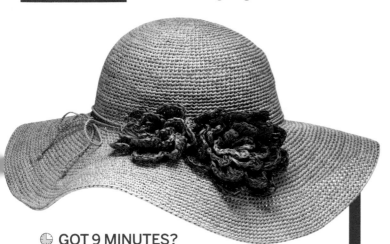

GOT 10 MINUTES?
Reduce the cost of your road trip

Gassing up for a long drive? No need to drive around town searching for the lowest price: Visit GasBuddy.com and enter your ZIP code or click on your state to find the best deal. Gas prices are higher in urban or affluent areas and at stations directly off the highway, the site says. Driving a few miles out of the way to refuel can pay off in savings.

GOT 12 MINUTES?
Hit the slopes off-season

For fantastic deals to some of the nation's prettiest resort towns, consider a spring or fall trip to a fancy ski resort. Chichi properties in Vail and Aspen, Colorado; Park City, Utah; and Stowe, Vermont, offer family-friendly activities such as horseback riding, mountain biking, hiking, zip lines, and outdoor concerts and movies. Summer hotel rates can be about half the price of winter rates and go even lower in spring and fall. You'll get all that après-hike charm, minus the crowds.

GOT 9 MINUTES?
Snag a fabulous beach place

JULY IS THE time for last-minute summer rental deals, says Christine Moore, an agent with Carlson GMAC Real Estate in Gloucester, Massachusetts. "By midmonth, owners with empty homes may drop prices 15 percent or more." How to connect with your dream cottage:

CAST A SMALL NET Instead of scratching your head at all the options, research an area and narrow your search to focus on only one or two towns that appeal to you.
MAKE CONTACT Ask the chamber of commerce to recommend a real estate agent who handles rentals in the area.
BE SPECIFIC Tell the agent what you are able to spend and how many rooms you want. Renting away from the waterfront could save you at least 10 percent. Ask the agent to e-mail photographs of suitable houses to you.
UNDERBID When making an offer, start below the asking price because owners may be willing to bargain late in the season. You can use the savings to splurge on another summer must-have that you can use when you return home, such as a backyard hammock or a brand-new grill.

GOT 2 MINUTES?
Crash a ritzy resort

Whenever you reserve a room in budget lodging, also book a massage at the nearest upscale resort. Spa guests are typically entitled to use the facilities all day long. Hello, hot tub!

GOT 30 SECONDS?
Grab an airline upgrade
To up your odds of jumping to first class for free, dress well (no sweats!) and tell agents you're game to be moved to a later flight if they're overbooked.

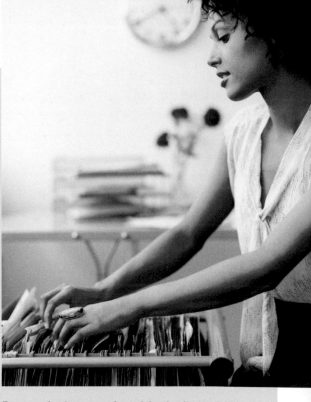

🕐 GOT 3 MINUTES?

Figure out if you need an accountant

Wondering if it's time to call in a tax pro? Answer the following questions.

Are your wages less than $100,000?
☐ Yes   ☐ No

Do you take the standard deduction?
☐ Yes   ☐ No

Can you claim few adjustments or credits?
☐ Yes   ☐ No

If you answered yes to all three, you may qualify for the IRS's simpler tax forms, 1040EZ or 1040A. If you answered no to any of them or if you answered yes only to the standard deduction question, keep going.

Do you have a computer and are you comfortable using tax software?
☐ Yes   ☐ No

Are your tax complications limited to common situations such as owning a home, itemizing deductions, investing in stocks and mutual funds or being self-employed?
☐ Yes   ☐ No

If you answered yes to both, you'll be fine using Intuit's TurboTax or H&R Block's TaxCut software. They'll lead you through the complicated forms, check that you don't miss a deduction and even provide help if you're audited. Answered no to either question? Keep going.

Do you feel uncomfortable dealing with your taxes or like to get input from an expert?
☐ Yes   ☐ No

Do you have any substantial tax complications such as investment real estate or a stake in a partnership?
☐ Yes   ☐ No

If you answered yes to either of these, find a tax professional, such as an accountant. You'll get more tailored advice and won't have to sort through complicated tax topics on your own. But remember: You still need to keep good tax records for your accountant throughout the year.

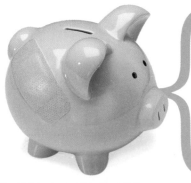

🕐 GOT 5 MINUTES?

Cut taxes on doctor bills

The next time you're allowed to update your workplace benefits package, see if you can get a flexible-spending account. FSAs let you set aside pretax money to cover health-related costs such as copayments and glasses, but only about 20 percent of employees take advantage of them. Yet paying with pretax funds automatically saves you 40 cents on the dollar. Think of it as a gift from the government!

⊕ GOT 5 MINUTES?
Earn credit for your clothes

YOU CAN CLEAR out your closets, donate the castoffs to charity and get a tax break. To do so, you'll need to itemize your deductions and keep receipts for everything you've donated. How much to take? Tax rules say you're allowed fair market value—but the place you've donated your goodies to isn't responsible for determining how much that is. Rather than estimating (or guessing) what those four shirts might sell for at a resale shop, use software like TurboTax ItsDeductible or H&R Block DeductionPro to figure it out. Donate more than $500 worth of items and you'll need to add an extra tax form (Form 8283) to your return.

⊕ GOT 2 MINUTES?
Get wise to itemizing

IN 2006, the standard deduction was $5,150 for singles and $10,300 for marrieds filing jointly. If you took it, you may have paid the IRS more than you needed to. That's because itemizers can write off home mortgage interest (a huge break for those who bought recently), state and local taxes (an especially big deal in high-tax states such as New York and California) and charitable donations, as well as a slew of smaller items (including the cost of preparing your taxes!). Even if you think it won't pay to itemize, plug the numbers into tax-prep software and see—you might be surprised.

⊕ GOT 10 MINUTES?
Turn losses into gains

IF YOU LOST money in the stock market this year, there is a silver lining. Once you've decided you'd rather not be invested in those losers anymore, dump them for a tax break. What's it worth? The tax law allows you to use this year's capital losses to offset the year's gains from other investments. Fill out a Schedule D form. Then use any remaining net capital loss to offset taxes on up to $3,000 of ordinary income, at which point the tax rates are higher. If you wind up with a larger net loss than you can use in a single year, roll over the remainder to reduce taxes on future returns.

⊕ GOT 15 MINUTES?
Purge your paperwork

Unless a taxpayer has committed fraud or substantially understated her income, the IRS has three years to conduct an audit. After that, you have the green light to toss most records related to previous-year tax returns. Keep any documents pertaining to the value of your home and those related to long-term investments you still own. If you claim a loss for worthless securities, you need to keep the paperwork for seven years.

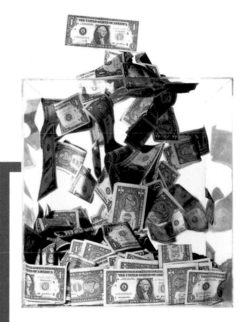

⊕ GOT 2 MINUTES?
Scrutinize your paycheck

Receiving a large refund feels great, but it means you're giving the IRS too much from every paycheck. You don't want the government sitting on cash you could be investing! To figure out your withholding number, go to the online calculator at IRS .gov and plug in your numbers. Recalculate if you buy a house or have a child.

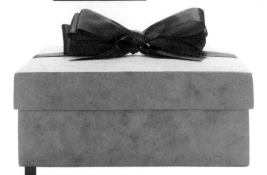

◷ GOT 4 MINUTES?
Learn how to give confidently

DESPITE OUR GOOD intentions, many of us write checks to charity haphazardly. Take these steps to help your pet causes—and add happiness to your own life, too.

PINPOINT YOUR PASSIONS The first question to ask is not How much can I afford to give? but What truly matters to me? Jot down three of your passions (e.g., the planet, curing cancer, educating kids). For each, decide:
- Do I want to give locally, nationally or internationally?
- Do I want to focus on the root causes of problems (for instance, organizations that work to end world hunger) or satisfy immediate needs (a soup kitchen)?
- Do I want to support large charities or smaller ones?

DECIDE HOW MUCH TO GIVE Technically, there is no right amount. "Basically, it's whatever makes you comfortable, but I like the idea of starting at 2 or 3 percent of your income a year, regardless of your salary," says Karen Altfest, a financial planner in New York City.

DIVIDE AND CONQUER Split your total yearly giving in three and direct those amounts to your three favorite causes. Or try one bigger gift and two smaller ones.

ALLOW FOR SPONTANEITY Set aside some funds for impulse donations. If nothing moves you to dash off a last-minute check or two, give the money to the cause you feel most connected to at the end of the year.

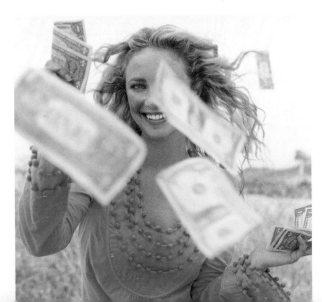

◷ GOT 10 MINUTES?
Be kind to strangers

Even if you're cash poor, you can still help out with these six ways to give:

Donate hours. In 2005, Americans volunteered about $280 billion worth of time. To find groups that need hands-on aid, go to VolunteerMatch.org.

Take a vacation. To make a far-flung impact, try GlobalVolunteers.org, which connects people with community-development projects and runs trips melding travel with volunteerism. (You pay your own airfare and a fee covering room, board and program expenses.)

Work up a sweat. Do yourself and others good by signing up to walk, run or bike for breast cancer, AIDS, multiple sclerosis or a wealth of other causes; get info at Active.com.

Find your phone a new home. Instead of stashing that outmoded mobile in your junk drawer, give it to either ShelterAlliance.net or WirelessFoundation.com. Both groups recycle old phones and also donate funds to victims of domestic violence.

Leggo that laptop. Go to TechSoup .org for low-income schools in your area that take used computers.

Give the gift of giving. At JustGive .org, you can buy a gift certificate for the charity of your recipient's choice. Getting married? Register for donations to your favorite causes. It sure beats another salad bowl.

YOUR MONEY TO-DON'T LIST

»Don't push for a huge salary in an interview; you'll be less likely to be hired. Negotiate after you get an offer.

»Don't spend your tax refund all at once. Use it to pay credit card debt, stock up your SOS fund or take a trip.

»Don't hastily shove money into your hairdresser's palm. Look her in the eye and say, "Thanks." Tipping gracefully is a sign of confidence.

»Don't pay a neighbor to shovel snow. Do it yourself and skip the gym.

»Don't make snap decisions about what stocks to buy and sell. Pick carefully and stick with your choices.

»Don't ask a man for money advice. A recent poll found women make fewer investing gaffes, partly because we tend to be more patient than men.

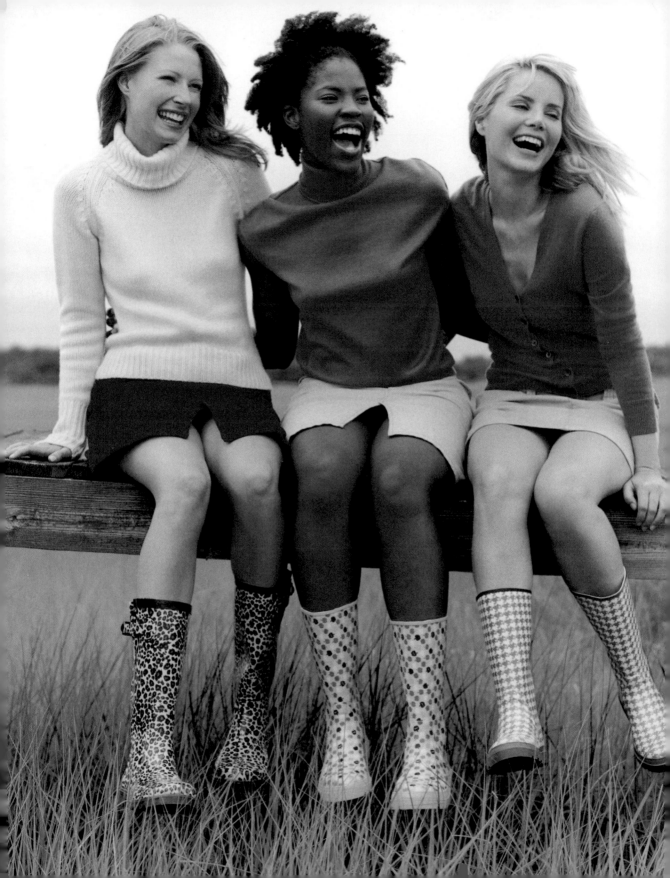

relationship rescues

A big part of living a full and rewarding life is having people to share it with. Use the tools in this chapter to build stronger bonds with those around you—friends and family, lovers, coworkers and even neighbors. You will find that your efforts are repaid a thousandfold because having close ties to others heightens your enjoyment of the good times and provides a soft landing if your spirits fall.

The only 10 things you need to know to make all of your relationships flourish

Wouldn't it be great if your family, friends and colleagues could always intuit exactly what you needed—and you always behaved perfectly toward everyone in your orbit? Nice fantasy. Truth is, put relationships on autopilot, and they may stall or crash. But invest some care, and they'll soar. Below are keys to creating harmony and community.

1 Assemble a support circle

There's a myth that happy people are pros at coping with things on their own. In fact, cheery folks know how to get guidance and support from others, so that in rocky times, they're well covered. Assemble your own emotional SWAT team by writing down what you most value in each of your friends (Irene's honesty, Sasha's sensitivity). You'll be better able to reach out on those occasions when you need it, and you won't depend on one person to shoulder all the weight. It really does take a village.

2 Seek role models

It's great to have pals who are going through the same life experiences you are, but it's also important to surround yourself with mentors who've already been where you're going. In a study of 700 people, Emmy Werner, Ph.D., developmental psychologist at the University of California at Davis, discovered that the most resilient women had, as young children, found people to look up to, such as teachers or grandparents. By the time these women reached adulthood, they had organized new mentor networks. So make a lunch date with a higher-up. Call your great-aunt. You'll find folks whose very existence reassures you that you are not alone in this world.

3 Live in the present

The average American spends almost five hours a day glued to the boob tube and countless more attached to a computer or BlackBerry.

Research shows when you watch TV, you're less apt to communicate or spend time with friends and family and more likely to feel dissatisfied. No wonder. TV's hunk of the month won't help you find Mr. Right or give you a shoulder to cry on; only flesh-and-blood loved ones can do that, so make them a priority. Don't eat family dinners with the TV on; never forgo plans with your pals to watch a show. And when you're with company, switch off your attention-grabbing gadgets so you can revel in the real-world love all around you.

4 Hone your communication skills

So much of the interplay in relationships takes place between the lines. Yes, what you say is important. Equally so is how you say it: the expression on your face as you speak to a colleague, the warmth in your voice when you chat on the phone with your mate, the light touch on your friend's arm as she tells you about her ailing dog. All of these nonverbal ways of communicating can have a huge impact on the quality of your day-to-day interactions. When you are mindful of the subtle cues you give off, you'll be more likely to have rewarding relationships.

5 Fight right

Arguments are inevitable in relationships, but if you know how to argue well, conflict can *improve* your bond. The key is to stay civil and follow some basic rules. When you're angry, discuss how you feel, not what the other person has done wrong. When someone has hurt you, indict the event, not the person's character. What not to do: give the silent treatment. Being ostracized triggers a reaction in the region of the brain that senses physical pain, experts at Purdue University in West Lafayette, Indiana, say. Go ahead and fight, but do it fairly and with respect.

6 Make peace with the past

Whom do you punish when you hold a grudge? The mother of your child's schoolmate who insulted you? The friend who betrayed you? Or yourself? Experts note that when you feel vengeful toward a person who has harmed you, *you* end up feeling unhappier. On the flip side, forgiving folks tend to be more satisfied and less depressed and anxious. Forgiveness is also associated with improved sleep and reduced symptoms of illness. So find resolution by recognizing how a painful experience has helped you grow. Then let go of your gripes and welcome joy.

7 Raise the stakes

When you're dealt a good hand in poker, you up the ante and hope the other players at the table see your raise and stay in the game. When life drops a new friend into your path, do the same. Raise the intimacy stakes by disclosing something about yourself, which in turn will prompt your friend (or mate) to do likewise. Then be a generous listener and let your new confidante know that you care about what she has to say. There's no better way to deepen a connection.

8 Keep it fresh

Variety is the spice of life—especially when it comes to relationships. Research has shown that new couples who do new and challenging activities together are more likely to remain close and committed over the long term. The same holds true for friends. Why? The more zing to your plans, the more appeal to your pals. So, mix it up. Take a knitting class together, plan a girlfriends' getaway to surf camp or throw a sex-toy party. You're not only spreading fun but also good health: Research has shown socializing can have as much of a positive impact on your health as quitting smoking, working out and eating right.

9 Be happy with yourself

The number-one thing you can do to better any relationship is improve your own state of mind. Research shows that happy people have closer and more satisfying relationships with friends, romantic partners and family members than unhappy people. (Though which comes first, the happiness or the solid bonds, is still unknown.) The contented folks also tend to be more agreeable and less neurotic than their unhappy counterparts. Look around at the links in your life. If you're always dissatisfied with friends (and everyone else), pay attention to what's actually going on with you. The more you work on your own happiness, the more you'll find it with others.

10 Say thank you

More than a matter of manners, a deep-hearted and sincere expression of gratitude can strengthen your relationships and make you happier. Expressing appreciation not only makes the recipient of your thanks feel good but also connects you to whatever beneficent act made you feel grateful in the first place. Write a thank-you letter to someone in your life who has made a profound difference but whom you've never properly thanked, and then read it out loud to that person. Doing so will put a smile on both of your faces.

⏲ GOT 4 MINUTES?
Learn how to act your age

If you still behave with your parents the way you did when you were a teenager, it's probably because your relationship with them is very much the way it was the day you went off to college—which leaves both sides stuck in old patterns. You can't change your parents, but you can alter the way you relate to them, then hope that they will reciprocate.

1 **DO UNTO YOUR FOLKS** Do you act the same way with your parents as you do with other adults in your life? For instance, have you ever stormed out of a girlfriend's house after she suggested the guy you were dating sounded like a jerk? Probably not. Start treating Mom and Dad with the warmth and respect you would give a friend. Even if they still nag, you'll feel better for behaving like the grown-up you now are.

2 **ZAP CONFLICT** It's helpful to tackle any of your ongoing arguments in a direct but nonconfrontational manner (the opposite of what you probably did as a teen). One good way to do this: Invite your folks to a neutral, public location such as a restaurant—where you'll be less apt to regress and have a meltdown—and say, "I've been feeling tension between us. Can we discuss it?" Then calmly say your piece.

3 **STOP BLAMING** Even if you didn't have the ideal childhood, now that you're an adult, it's time to take responsibility for your life's circumstances and for your feelings. Do this by expressing troubles with "I" statements: "I've been struggling with how to deal with this problem." If you find yourself becoming combative, hit PAUSE. ("I'm having trouble expressing myself without getting emotional. Let's talk about this another time.") Set a definite date to meet again.

4 **ADJUST YOUR EXPECTATIONS** It's tough to give up the idea of having perfect parents, but part of growing up is realizing that Mom and Dad are only human. Once you accept this fact and stop expecting your folks to be infallible superheroes, you'll be more able to work around their limitations and focus on the good in your relationship.

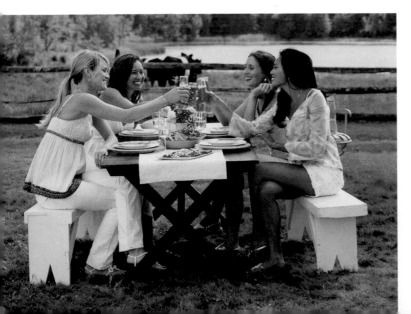

⏲ GOT 15 MINUTES?
Set up a sibling dinner

Once upon a time they drove you crazy, but these days, your sisters and brothers are your closest allies. Staying connected to them, by, say, having a monthly potluck, is good for you. Domestic routines such as family meals are linked to well-being and stronger relationships, the *Journal of Family Psychology* reports. "There are few better remedies for unhappiness than nurturing a bond with people who care deeply about you," says David Myers, Ph.D., professor of psychology at Hope College in Holland, Michigan. Pass the pasta.

◷ GOT 10 MINUTES? Tame a meddlesome mom

She calls five times a day. She bugs you to get married. She offers unhelpful advice. Try these tricks to assert your adulthood.

SHE SAYS	YOU SAY
"Where did your date take you? Did he kiss you good-night?"	"I love you, Mom, but I'd like to keep that private." It's likely that your mother simply wants to be included in your life, so share a tidbit of office gossip or ask her for a recipe.
"I know I've called you four times today, but…"	Absolutely nothing. Let her call go straight to voice mail, and then call back when it's convenient for you. And when you wrap up your next conversation, schedule a day and time to chat.
"You need to discipline your kids or they'll get spoiled."	"I'd prefer not to discuss how we discipline the children right now." Though you may feel like telling her to zip it, both of you will feel better if you can manage to keep your cool even as you firmly imply she should butt out.

◷ GOT 5 MINUTES?

Appreciate your in-laws They're part of the package deal you got when you married your mate and, no, they're not returnable. But the new clan, even if difficult, still has things you can relish. You'll gain…

INSIGHT INTO YOUR SPOUSE Not only will you learn where he got his eyes or sense of humor but you'll also hear stories of his childhood that he's long forgotten.

ALL THE FUN FAMILY LORE When your kids ask, "How did Grandma and Grandpa meet?" you can tell them, because you'll have heard the amusing tales firsthand.

A MORE DETAILED HEALTH HISTORY Because so many medical conditions are inherited, it can help to get the complete picture of what runs in his family.

MORE PEOPLE TO LOVE—and more people to love you, too. Who doesn't need lots of affection? Ponder this thought the next time your mother-in-law nags you.

GOT 15 MINUTES?
Build a friend web

Not every pal is destined to become your lifelong soulmate, supporting you through work and relationship crises alike. It makes more sense to be able to rely on a wide variety of different people to fill the many kinds of needs in your life. The benefit? You'll be less likely to make unrealistic demands on any one person. Here are the five most important friends for you to include in your circle.

THE OLD FRIEND	THE EVENT FRIEND	THE BOSOM BUDDY	THE WORK PAL	THE CASUAL FRIEND
No matter how different you may be now, she knows about all the skeletons in your closet—your Goth phase, the guy you lost your virginity to—and loves you anyway. There's great comfort in that.	Whether it's a new Cézanne retrospective at the art museum or the opening of a fancy nightclub, this friend is your go-to girl for socializing, able to be good company in a variety of social settings.	It's two in the morning and you just read an e-mail informing you that your ex-boyfriend is engaged. This friend is the one who will race over to your apartment, let you sob on her shoulder, then tuck you in to bed.	You and your boss are butting heads about how to deal with a new client, and you don't know what to do. Your work pal is the objective insider who can help you strategize about career issues.	You two may not have tons in common, but she's always up for sharing a last-minute drink or flick or joining you for a run in the park. Keep her on speed dial for times when you need company.

GOT 15 MINUTES?
Spice up Saturday

Break out of the dinner-and-a-movie monotony and arrange one of these offbeat activities with your friends. **Go floral.** Call a local flower shop and ask the designer to teach you how to make your own eye-popping bouquets. **Plan a grape escape.** See if your favorite wine shop will dispatch a sommelier to your house for a tasting lesson. **Get in stitches.** Ask that hip chick at the fancy yarn store to conduct a private knitting lesson for you and your buds. **Schedule a roving dinner.** Set up a traveling supper party, with each person hosting a different course at her house. If you have more friends than courses, have some bring wine pairings to each. Remember to designate drivers.

GOT 10 MINUTES?
Adapt your relationship

Just because a friend moved, got married or had a baby doesn't mean an end to the relationship. Simply make some adjustments. If you used to get together at a restaurant for drinks and dinner every Thursday like clockwork, try setting up monthly visits or even regular phone dates. Be flexible, and allow your relationship to evolve as your lives evolve, and you may find yourselves growing even closer.

◷ GOT 15 MINUTES?

Plan the ultimate girlfriend getaway

Taking a trip with your best buddy can be incredibly bonding—or incredibly fraught if you have different ideas of fun. We make it easy with trips that will appeal to you both.

SHE WANTS	YOU WANT	WHERE TO GO
Peace and quiet	To party	The Marquis Los Cabos (MarquisLosCabos.com), a Mexican beachfront resort midway between the party town of Cabo San Lucas and the artsy village of San José del Cabo. By day, hang out at the infinity pools or visit the Spa Marquis. At night, hit the dance clubs in Cabo San Lucas or the cozy eateries of traditional San José.
Natural wonders	Very few tourists	At the vast, uncrowded Redwood National and State Parks in Northern California, you'll both be awed by the majesty of the giant redwood trees—and the feeling of having them all to yourself. Camp beneath the conifers, or refresh at the Victorian Carter House Inns in Eureka (CarterHouse.com).
Hard-core adventure	Ancient culture	Head South to Peru's national treasure, Machu Picchu. The guides at Mountain Travel Sobek (MtSobek.com) offer hikes around the awe-inspiring Incan citadel that range from strenuous itineraries through icy glaciers to beginner's visits that feel like little more than a walk in the park.
Luxe digs	Great skiing	The tiny village of Zermatt at the base of Switzerland's Matterhorn is famous for its hiking and its long ski season. Stay at the luxurious chalet-style Romantik Hotel Julen (www.zermatt.ch/julen/e/hotel.html) and enjoy snowshoeing, snowboarding, mountain biking and more. Come dusk, don heels and experience an après-ski scene that makes Aspen look quaint.

🕐 GOT 4 MINUTES?

Dazzle every man you meet There truly never is a second chance to make a first impression. Avoid these common pitfalls with scientifically proven tactics.

What not to do	What to do instead
Avert your eyes. Peering away from a hot guy could leave him thinking you're not excited about getting to know him.	**Lock eyes.** Experts believe that a direct gaze triggers a response in the brain region associated with anticipation of pleasure. Making eye contact is also associated with attractiveness.
Stifle a smile. When you meet someone you like, resist the temptation to play it cool, even if you feel like a grinning idiot.	**Say cheese.** Research shows that when you smile, even if it's forced, the tiny changes in muscle groupings create a more positive brain state for both you and the person you're beaming at.
Divide your attention. Focus on the person you're with. Acting interested in everyone and everything can be a turn-off.	**Be picky.** A study of speed daters in *Psychological Science* found that those who were seeking the most potential suitors were more likely to be rejected than folks who preferred only a few.
Overshare. Although you may think you're being open, talking about yourself too much, too soon can be overkill.	**Perk up your ears.** Studies have shown the more you listen to someone you're meeting for the first time, the more your attention will eventually be returned. So be patient. Your chance will come.

🕐 GOT 2 MINUTES? **Find out if you belong together**

Evaluate your bond by checking true or false for the following statements.

He makes you feel like a million bucks.

☐ True ☐ False

In a strong union, both partners are at their best in each other's company. Can't tell if this is the case? Ask your friends if the guy you're seeing brings out the qualities they most cherish in you.

You each savor your solo time.

☐ True ☐ False

If you relish your solitude and he enjoys his, too, it's a sign your bond is healthy. Couples should complement each other, not be joined at the hip. The stronger your sense of self, the more you'll bring to your twosome.

Part of you loves him; another part doesn't.

☐ True ☐ False

You either love someone or you don't; there's no ambivalence when it comes to the real thing. Of course there will be times when your man makes you fume, but your essential feelings of love should stay intact.

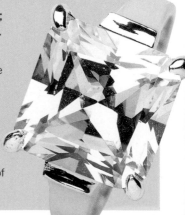

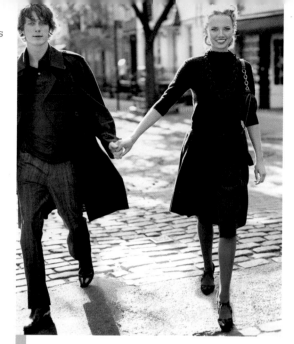

🕐 GOT 12 MINUTES?
Stoke long-distance love

Try these little communication tips to help bridge the divide with your faraway sweetie.

- Be boring. To stay connected, share the mundane stuff, like what happened at work.
- Unload a little. Hiding your troubles will weaken your bond and create distance.
- Titillate. Keep desire strong with phone sex. Too shy? Send a racy text message.
- Plan your next rendezvous. Be clear about when you'll see each other in person again.

🕐 GOT 10 MINUTES?
Let him down
Tips to ease a breakup for both of you

PUT YOURSELF IN HIS PLACE Pondering what it would be like to hear what you're telling him will help you break the news more gently.

BE HONEST—TO A POINT No need to announce you're dumping him because he's a bore. Couch it by saying something general such as, "Our styles are different."

BE CONSTRUCTIVE, NOT CRITICAL Instead of "I'm sick of always hearing you talk about yourself," try "Sometimes it feels as if you're not interested in what I say."

EMPHASIZE THE POSITIVE Even if he's done something wrong, show appreciation rather than devaluing the whole experience.

🕐 GOT 1 MINUTE?
Get all touchy-feely

When you're in the throes of new love, don't feel shy about cuddling. Not only does holding hands with your sweetie reduce stress, but research also shows that hugging optimizes the flow of mood-enhancing chemicals oxytocin and serotonin, which have been found to promote bonding. For best results, squeeze your squeeze for a minimum of six seconds.

🕐 GOT 10 MINUTES? Handle rejection

You thought that first date went great, but he declined to go out again. Here's how to move on:

- Don't take it too personally. Rather than worrying that he thinks you're unattractive, remind yourself that there are many reasons (work, his ex) for his not wanting to continue things.
- Get a reality check. Talk to friends who can reassure you of how wonderful you are.
- Garner support. Holing up to lick your wounds after a rejection will only make things worse. Reach for the phone: Enjoying support and love from others can greatly improve your mood.
- Never give up. This time you were rejected. Let it go and you'll soon be back on track.

⏱ GOT 2 MINUTES?

Make nice When people behave passive-aggressively, it can be tempting to hit back hard. But you'll resolve the situation faster and feel happier if you remain civil and nip the stealth attack in the bud.

Hostile move	How to deal
A buddy bad-mouths you to mutual friends behind your back.	Don't lash out—you risk exacerbating the gossip. Instead, say, "I've heard you're mad at me. I'd like to know why." Whether she backs off, airs her beefs or denies it, you're apt to feel better by having taken control of the situation.
Your assistant always "forgets" to give you phone messages.	Instead of laying blame, which may make her defensive, ask her to suggest an improved message system. People tend to be passive-aggressive when they feel powerless. By giving her choices, you'll make her feel more autonomous.
A neighbor sweeps trash onto your lawn.	Don't sweep it back. Ask your neighbor an open question: "Do you know how that garbage got there?" By inviting conversation, you can discover the true reason for the sweeping, and together, you can work toward a resolution.

⏱ GOT 5 MINUTES? Sidestep a lovers' spat

Things are bound to get rocky with your mate now and again, but not every disagreement has to lead to all-out war. Use these strategies in your day-to-day interactions and you may well head off a heated showdown.

Practice random acts of kindness. Showing little examples of appreciation such as offering an unsolicited back massage can add up exponentially.

Listen to yourself talk to your mate. Pay attention to your tone. Is it critical? Do your requests sound as if you are criticizing him? If so, soften your voice.

Be nice when you begin a big talk. You should be civil even when you're not feeling especially nice. Doing so will set the tone for your entire exchange.

Invite your partner out for a walk. When things are getting tense, a change of scenery can often help the two of you avoid rehashing the same old arguments.

Excuse yourself from the room. If your temper rises during discussions with your mate, take a break until you can speak calmly and productively.

⊕ GOT 12 MINUTES? **Resolve conflict quicker**

Think back to your last major quarrel. You probably recall the feelings, but you may be a little fuzzy on what set off the tiff in the first place. Truth is, how we fight is often more important than what we fight about. "Ideally, the act of arguing should foster closeness," says Deborah Cox, Ph.D., associate professor of counseling and gender studies at Missouri State University at Springfield. Try these rules of engagement.

Raise a ruckus. Don't be afraid to make noise. "Arguing loudly isn't in itself a bad idea," especially if that's your natural instinct, Cox says. "It's important for the object of your rage to know you're really mad." Plus, a study at the University of Aberdeen in Scotland found that women who suppress their irate emotions end up feeling even more furious. But steer clear of hurling insults, which erode intimacy long-term.

Own your emotions. Conflicts that kick off with "you" statements ("You are so selfish!") are more apt to spiral out of control or end in stony silence. Instead, acknowledge responsibility for your feelings with "I" statements, as in "I feel as if you're not thinking of me." Making yourself vulnerable suggests you're open to hearing what your partner is thinking, too.

Make a concession. Even if you're convinced you're right, giving in on even a minor point can make the clash less combative, Cox says. If your mate is steamed that you forgot to give him a phone message, for instance, don't snap; say something like, "I understand you're nervous about your big meeting." Then remind him that you're doing the best you can.

Write it out. If your talk starts to turn nasty, try saying, "I want to discuss this, but not this way." Then excuse yourself for a few minutes and jot down what you wish you could spew, Cox advises. ("I feel like your servant when you expect me to run your errands.") Once your emotions are on paper and you're no longer in the heat of the moment, it can be easier to gain perspective and come up with solutions. Then let the talks finish and the making up begin!

Drop your megaphone. If your mate is upset with you about something, close your mouth and listen for 10 whole minutes before you launch into your defense. Fully focusing on your partner's words— no interrupting allowed—breeds compassion and respect and may well melt his ire.

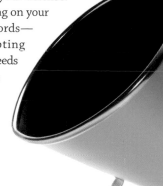

⊕ GOT 10 MINUTES?
Plan an escape

Even when you and your sweetie are having a rough patch, plan weekly dates for uninterrupted talk time and quarterly romantic getaways—no kids in tow. You'll be amazed how this time alone together can replenish you and energize your relationship.

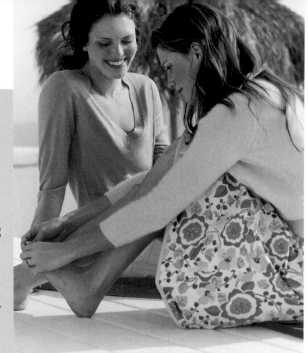

🕐 GOT 3 MINUTES?

Don't take it personally

How many squabbles arise from a tendency to personalize other people's actions or moods? Here's how to stop making it about you and put an end to petty gripes caused by oversensitivity for good.

The dis	You think	The depersonalized reaction
Your friend cancels your dinner date at the last minute.	"She must not value me. That's the last time I make plans with her!"	Be empathetic to what's happening in her life. Maybe she has troubles at home or is overwhelmed by her work. Ask if you can do anything to help. Even if you can't, you'll feel better for having offered.
Your grumpy mate refuses to chat.	"He must be mad at me, and I'll find out why, come hell or high water."	Turn on CNN. Watch 10 minutes of news about wars, hurricanes, etc. Are those your fault? Nope. So why assume his mood is your doing? Back off, and let him stew in peace. He'll come around soon.
Your boss is mum about the proposal you wrote.	"She clearly thinks it stinks. What the hell does she know, anyhow?"	Analyze why you're so worried about her reaction. Maybe you doubt that your proposal is up to snuff. If that's the case, it's time to raise your own bar so you can be more confident about your work.

⊕ GOT 1 MINUTE?
Customize your mea culpa

Stow this away in the Men and Women Are From Different Planets file. Research shows that we tend to react to apologies differently. So learn how to tailor your sorries to the sexes.

WOMEN tend to want an acknowledgment of what they're going through and how they're feeling. If you were bitchy on the phone to your pal, say, "I know I made you feel bad when I snapped at you on the phone. I'm really sorry about that."

MEN often aren't interested in knowing that you feel their pain. In fact, your sympathy may actually make guys feel more vulnerable and worse. If you pissed off your date by accidentally blabbing some confidential info about him to a friend, don't bother telling him how betrayed you know he must feel. Instead, stick to a matter-of-fact apology. Say, "I'm sorry I was so indiscreet, and I'll make sure it doesn't happen again."

GOT 30 SECONDS?
Make up before bed
If you and your mate have a P.M. fight, de-escalate before turning off the lights, even if you only agree to disagree until the morning.

⊕ GOT 5 MINUTES? Release old hurts

Studies have shown that holding a grudge can lead to stress and unhappiness, whereas forgiveness can have the opposite effect. But just because you forgive someone who hurt you doesn't mean you need to reconcile with him; in some cases it may be healthier not to. Remember, the forgiveness is mostly for your benefit and peace of mind. Follow these steps to move on and feel happier.

PURGE THE FRUSTRATION Tell your story of woe to a few close friends. This will help you explore your feelings about the rift and obtain a sense of perspective.

WRITE A "LET IT ALL OUT" LETTER Rant and rave about everything that's bothering you. Read what you've written out loud in private. Then, instead of sending it, burn it in your kitchen sink, imagining your pain going up in smoke.

BREATHE IN CALM The next time you think about what happened, decouple your body's automatic stress response from your memory of the hurtful event. Instead of tensing up or starting in on an inner rant, inhale and exhale deeply or relax in any way you like.

RECAST YOUR STORY Victims don't have control of their life; heroes do. So make yourself the hero of your own saga. Think of it this way: Although someone else may have precipitated your misery, whether you stay miserable is up to you. You get to determine what you feel.

FOCUS ON WHAT'S IN IT FOR YOU Grudges can be hard to let go—after all, why should you do the pardoning when you were wronged? Remind yourself that forgiving can free you to move on with your life and reduce angst. After all, living well is the best revenge.

GOT 7 MINUTES?
Deal with a chronically late pal

Getting irritated with a perpetual late bird won't help, but these tips might.

1 WAIT PRODUCTIVELY Rather than stew, make the most of a toe-tapping session by reading an article that you've torn out. Or get rid of all the old receipts and dusty mints from your purse. The cathartic purging will do wonders for your handbag—and your mood.

2 ASSERT YOURSELF If the tardy person hasn't arrived 5 minutes before the movie is due to start, call her cell and say you've gone in and will save her a seat. Doing this beats getting angry and missing the trailers.

3 TRICK HER The next time you make a date, tell her to meet you at an offbeat time, such as 7:23. The specific and memorable number will make her think there's a reason to be prompt.

4 SHOW BY EXAMPLE To ensure your own on-time arrival, plan to be a few minutes early and bring an extra task to do when you get there, instead of trying to finish everything before you head out.

GOT 30 SECONDS?
Send an RSVP
Always respond to an invitation, even if it's only to say, "Sorry, can't make it. I'm busy that night." A nonresponse doesn't equal a decline.

GOT 15 MINUTES?
Pick a card, any card

The next time you're in a card shop, buy an assortment all at once, stamp them immediately and toss them in your purse. That way, it will be easy to send off a quick thank-you note or a thinking-of-you missive to a friend.

GOT 1 MINUTE?
Ace an intro

When introducing two strangers, break the ice by including some little tidbit such as, "Mike, this is Sandra. She just got back from climbing Mt. McKinley." That way, you'll give them something to talk about. If you ever find yourself introducing someone to an acquaintance whose name you've forgotten, no need to fumble. Simply say, "Hey. Great to see you. Have you met Sandra before?" To which the nameless one replies, "Not yet. I'm Bill," thus solving the mystery for you both.

⏱ GOT 5 MINUTES? Write the perfect thank-you

In this era of abbreviated, acronym-filled e-mail and text messages, a handwritten card can carry more meaning than ever. In case you've forgotten how to write one, here's a refresher course on dashing off a thank-you for three key occasions.

TO THANK A FRIEND FOR GOING ABOVE AND BEYOND FOR YOU

Dear Sara: I can't thank you enough for making my moving day go so smoothly. I was stressing—until you volunteered to pack my books.[1] I can't believe we unearthed my high school yearbook![2] Next time you move or want help with spring-cleaning, I'm your girl.[3] In the meantime, here's a gift certificate for a manicure to repair your thrashed nails.[4]

[1] Reflect on how your friend's act helped you by mentioning the act of kindness you're thanking her for directly. [2] Include a personal detail from the event to emphasize your sincerity. [3] Offer to return the favor. [4] If it's appropriate and if the spirit moves you, include a gift or token of your appreciation. When you need her again, she'll be there!

TO THANK YOUR HOSTESS FOR A WEEKEND STAY AT HER VACATION HOME

Dear Gail: Many thanks for this past weekend at your beautiful cottage.[1] Watching the sun rise from my comfy bed while sipping your delicious coffee was pure heaven.[2] Of course, the next day I didn't get up quite so early. I'm so sorry I slept through brunch.[3] Thank you again for your generous hospitality. Looking forward to seeing you soon.

[1] You'll want to send your missive quickly before the weekend fades, so write down the street address while you're there. [2] During your stay, record a few amusing moments so you can include specific details about the weekend. [3] Part of being a good guest is acknowledging the occasional faux pas, so don't be shy about owning up.

TO THANK A PROSPECTIVE EMPLOYER AFTER A JOB INTERVIEW

Dear Ms. Ellison: Thank you for taking the time to meet with me and to discuss the new direction of ACME Unlimited today.[1] Your analysis of the changing market dynamics was insightful.[2] Having worked abroad, I have a unique handle on the global marketplace, and I believe I can help ACME expand in this arena.[3] I look forward to hearing from you this week, and I'm available for any other questions you may have.[4]

[1] Be sure to send notes ASAP to everyone involved in the interview process—down to the assistant who made the arrangements. Double-check that you've spelled names right. [2] Cite some personal contribution the person made in the interview. [3] Briefly restate one point of your position. [4] Close with positive anticipation for your future.

⏱ GOT 15 MINUTES? Clean up your online image

YOUR BLIND DATE isn't the only one who is Googling you: According to a survey by ExecuNet, a head-hunting firm in Norwalk, Connecticut, 77 percent of recruiters troll the Internet for morsels on job candidates and 35 percent have eliminated people based on what they've found. Here's how to create a great online impression.

Keep tabs on yourself. Regularly type your name into several search engines to see what appears. If your college-era blog about your drunken spring break in Mexico pops up on the first page, you've got some online rehabbing to do.
Hit DELETE. If you find unflattering content, don't panic. Simply send a polite message to the site's webmaster explaining why the entry is potentially damaging and requesting that it be taken down. Most people will comply.
Create flattering content. Start by joining professional communities online (try LinkedIn.com or ZoomInfo.com), and update your stats often. Feeling more ambitious? Upgrade your virtual presence by acting virtuously off-line. Apply your talents to a philanthropic cause. You'll build a knock-their-socks-off Web ID, spread good karma and impress would-be employers with your good deeds and networking skills.

⏱ GOT 12 MINUTES?
Woo everyone in your office orbit

To shine at work, you don't only need to please your boss; you also have to make those under you happy. And in the best-case scenario, you'll do both at one time.

THE SITUATION	MANAGE UP	MANAGE DOWN
Your boss hands your team an important last-minute project.	Be upbeat and positive but also clear about any help you'll need: "That sounds great! Of course, we'll need to sideline low-priority projects and hire a temp to meet the deadline."	Acknowledge the extra work, but stress how it might lead to new opportunities and benefits (handing off less interesting work; a bonus).
You lose a major client after making a presentation.	Restore the boss's confidence by showing what you've learned from the fiasco. Explain what you'll do to prevent it from happening again.	Shoulder the blame and focus on bouncing back. Claiming responsibility shows your staff you're not looking for scapegoats. This, in turn, calms their fears.
An ambitious staffer takes credit for an idea that isn't hers.	Don't compete for kudos with underlings. Bosses hate dealing with pettiness. Your only option is to be professional and grin and bear it.	Don't punish the attention seeker; you'll only risk alienating her. To head off power plays like this in the future, give your best staffers credit as often as possible.

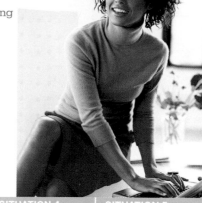

⊕ GOT 2 MINUTES?
Be e-mail smart Review this list of potential e-mail gaffes before you hit SEND to protect your reputation at work.

SITUATION 1	SITUATION 2	SITUATION 3	SITUATION 4	SITUATION 5
You respond to a coworker's note that her kid is selling Girl Scout cookies with "Fat thighs be damned, sign me up for 10 boxes of those Thin Mints."	Your supervisor announced a reduction in this year's bonuses. You write back, "You don't seem to have any idea how hard I work!"	You invite your business buddies to a party and put all their addresses in the "To" field.	You want your coworker to pass along contact info for a client, and you also want to catch up with her after the long weekend. You title the e-mail "Hi!"	You want your boss to know how happy you were with the results of your lunch meeting. So you write, "Hi there! ;-) The meeting went well! :-)"
Infraction You hit the REPLY ALL button, so the whole office got your order.	**Infraction** TWA (typing while angry)	**Infraction** Violating their privacy by sharing addresses of people who don't necessarily know one another.	**Infraction** Slapping on a vague subject line	**Infraction** Overusing emoticons
Click smart Start a fresh note to the senders of mass e-mails.	**Click smart** Save your missive as a draft until you've cooled off (at which point you'll want to do a thorough edit).	**Click smart** It's safe to assume that not all of your recipients want their info revealed. Use "bcc" instead.	**Click smart** Be clear about your message's content: "Wanda's contact info" or "Lunch today?"	**Click smart** Write clearly, using full sentences. Skip happy faces and other symbols.

⊕ GOT 3 MINUTES?
Ward off a coworker's bad attitude

Use these tactics to preempt the downer effect of a grumpy colleague.

- **SYMPATHIZE, DON'T EMPATHIZE** It's fine to be caring, but if you overidentify with someone's bad mood, you're inclined to inherit it.
- **MAINTAIN A STRAIGHT FACE** We're hardwired to mimic other people's expressions or tones of voice. But copy an irritated visage, and you might end up feeling prickly, too. Keep your face, voice and body language neutral when conversing with a grouch and you'll stay happy.
- **CHECK YOUR TEMPERATURE** After an encounter with an unhappy officemate, see how you feel. If you're suddenly angry, you may have "caught" a case of bad vibes. Let them go, and carry on your merry way.

⊕ GOT 1 MINUTE?

Read faces Use this crib sheet to understand the secret messages others are sending and to become more conscious of the statement your own face is making.

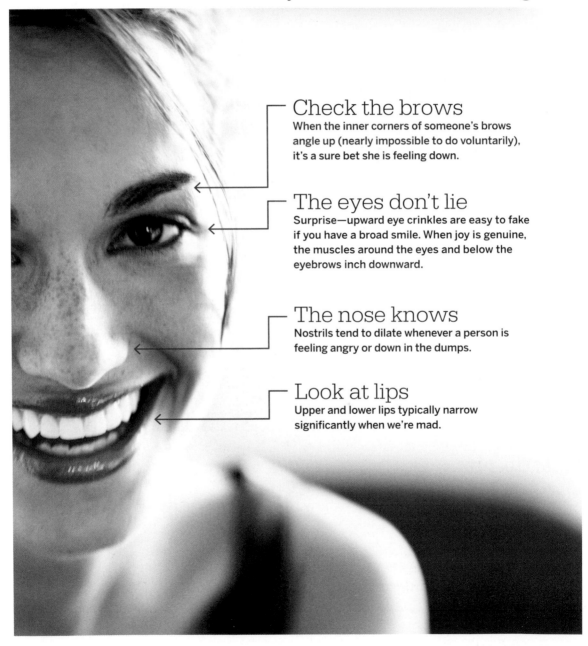

Check the brows
When the inner corners of someone's brows angle up (nearly impossible to do voluntarily), it's a sure bet she is feeling down.

The eyes don't lie
Surprise—upward eye crinkles are easy to fake if you have a broad smile. When joy is genuine, the muscles around the eyes and below the eyebrows inch downward.

The nose knows
Nostrils tend to dilate whenever a person is feeling angry or down in the dumps.

Look at lips
Upper and lower lips typically narrow significantly when we're mad.

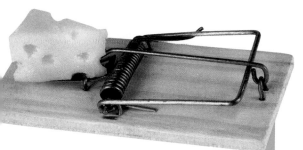

⏱ GOT 3 MINUTES?
Shake off someone

At every social event, there's the one person who traps you in a corner. To get unstuck, introduce the person to someone else you know. Nobody handy? Say, "Why don't we go meet some more people?" Then, after a few minutes of conversation, excuse yourself. If all else fails, say, "Pardon me, but there's someone I need to speak to. I'll try to catch up with you later." Don't feel bad. Mingling is what parties are about.

⏱ GOT 1 MINUTE?
Win over anyone

Just flash them a million-dollar grin. Chances are, they won't be able to help beaming back, according to a study in *Cognition and Emotion.* Scientists found that when volunteers were asked to scowl at happy faces, they had trouble making their mouth obey. It turns out that joy is contagious, so go ahead and spread some happiness, why don't you?

⏱ GOT 4 MINUTES?
Turn yourself into a social butterfly

Find shindigs stressful? Practice these meeting and mingling tips and you'll be the life of the party at your next fête.

PARTY PANIC	EASY FIX
I won't know anybody.	Head to the kitchen or bar. Revelers flock to both spots, so it will be a cinch to strike up a conversation. Avoid no-man's land: the couch.
I'll be underdressed/overdressed.	Call the host to ask what's appropriate. Or err on the side of formal. No one is going to fault you for looking too glam.
I'll have nothing to say.	Ask questions. ("I'm planning a European vacation. Have any suggestions?") People love giving opinions. Avoid polarizing topics.
I'll be bored to tears.	If the bash is a bust, ask the bartender to create a fun drink, name it after the host and show everyone how to make it. You'll mix things up.
I won't sound smart enough.	Read at least one section of the paper before you leave home. You'll find a fun nugget that you can impress the room with.

🕐 GOT 7 MINUTES?

Say it with flowers Different buds symbolize different sentiments. Let the guide below inspire you to communicate something special for each occasion.

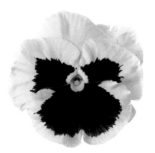

ZINNIA Says "I'm thinking of you even though you're far away"
GIVE TO An old friend

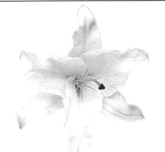

PANSY Named for the French word for thought; implies caring
GIVE TO A party hostess

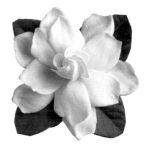

GARDENIA In Chinese tradition, this represents feminine grace
GIVE TO Your mother or sister

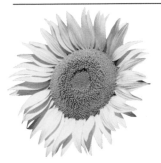

SUNFLOWER Ancient Incas placed this flower's image in their temples.
GIVE TO A pal who's been devoted

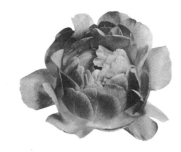

LILY Roman mythology holds that lilies grew from Juno's breast milk.
GIVE TO A new mother

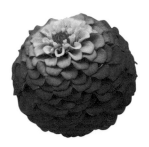

PEONY Named after Paeon, physician to the Greek gods
GIVE TO A sick friend

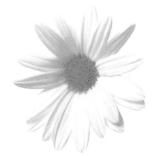

DAISY The official flower of April connotes youthful innocence.
GIVE TO Your favorite niece

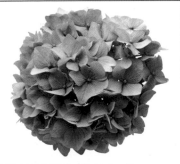

HYDRANGEA In Victorian times, these symbolized bragging rights.
GIVE TO A promoted coworker

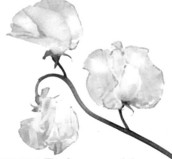

SWEET PEA The fragrance of these flowers lasts a long time.
GIVE TO Someone who is moving

YOUR RELATIONSHIP TO-DON'T LIST

»Don't feign sleep on a plane. Chance encounters are meaningful.

»Don't bring your BlackBerry with you to social occasions. Focus on the people you're with; e-mail can wait.

»Don't repeat yourself. Once you state your case in an argument, be quiet and give the other person some time to ponder your brilliance.

»Don't be the plan maker every Saturday. Change your routine: Let your sweetie plot out some evenings.

»Don't stress over holiday office gifts. Instead, send cards to show you donated your gift budget to charity.

»Don't ruminate about your ex. Doing so can reduce brain activity in regions linked to motivation. Smile by thinking about loved ones instead.

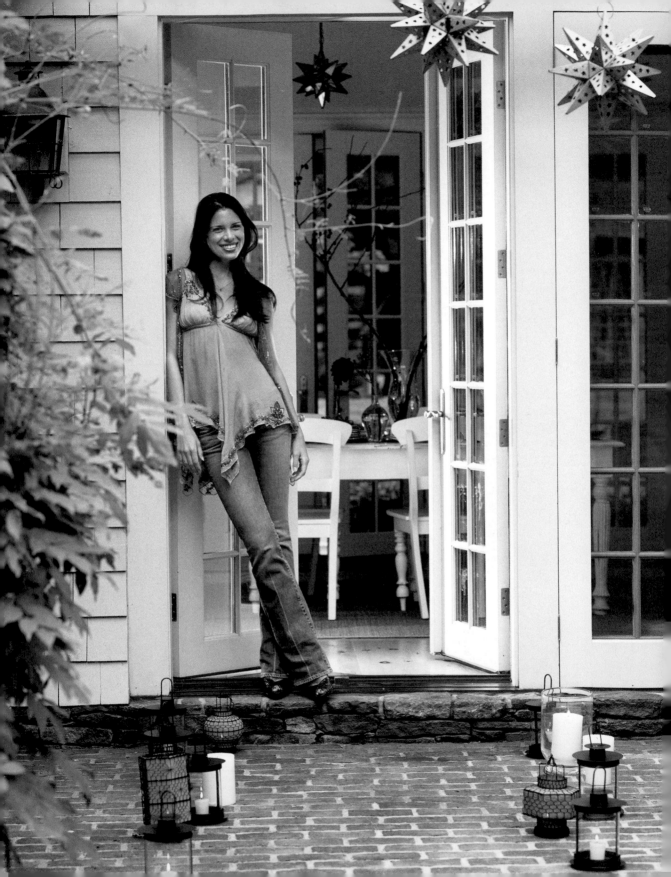

home makeovers

Transform your living space into a happier place with these inexpensive, easy design tips. You'll learn how to rearrange your living room so it feels instantly welcoming and how to choose paint colors effortlessly; you'll also find a foolproof trick to throwing together a last-minute celebration for 5 or 50. Your home will look and feel better inside and out and, as a result, so will you.

The only 10 things you need to know to turn your home into your very own haven

In our hurried, harried life, the best place to rejuvenate is the place you spend time in every day: your home. SELF's decorating principles will help you transform your dwelling into a refuge from life's craziness. And don't worry, you don't need an interior designer, 10,000 square feet or an obscenely large disposable income to get that there's-no-place-like-home feeling. Haven, here you come!

1 Parade your personality

Sure, re-creating a page out of a decorating magazine makes a pretty room, but if the stuff in it doesn't resonate with you, the space, no matter how posh, will end up feeling generic. When planning a room, focus more on how you want to feel in it and less on how you want it to look. Choose colors, textures and objects that evoke positive memories—for instance, a mirror decorated in beach glass you collected on Cape Cod or a rug you snagged on your trip to Istanbul. "Surrounding yourself with meaningful items gives you a sense of rootedness," says Erinn McGurn, a designer in New York City.

2 Make it human-centered

Just because you have a large and lovely TV, even one that is a flat-screen, that doesn't mean you and all your guests should have to stare at it 24/7. Friends aren't going to feel all the love in the room if they sense that you prioritize playthings over people. Tuck technology away into cabinets or corners, and encourage talk to flow freely by arranging furniture into conversation-fostering clusters—two chairs and a settee—within easy talking distance.

3 Lighten things up

Regardless of how much natural sunlight you get, every room should also have at least three additional sources of illumination, says Maxwell Gillingham-Ryan, interior designer and founder of ApartmentTherapy.com in New York City. Of those, very few should be ceiling lights because they tend to flatten out a space, making everyone look pasty. Add a few lamps with dimmers. Altering your lighting to suit your task or mood can give you a sense of peace by reinforcing the idea that you are in control.

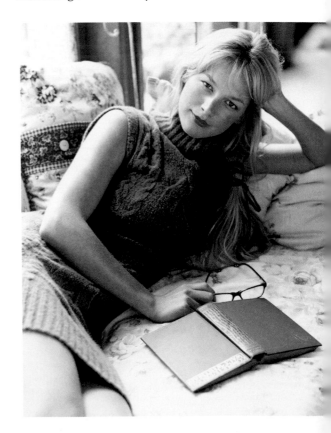

4 Carve out nooks and crannies

In every room, create cozy enclaves, each designed for a different activity. Start by thinking about what you want to do in a space—reflect, nap, play games, read. Then designate at least three uniquely inviting activity areas, such as a couch for lounging, a table and chair for working, two seats facing each other for talking. Ideally, all of them should be visible from the entrance so you can choose where to go. Lay rugs or set up privacy screens to define borders, and hang mirrors to add depth. The goal: Make every room feel both full of prospect yet intimate.

5 Edit your accessories

Sure, it's comforting to keep memories close at hand, but it's also important not to smother yourself with them; too many turn to clutter. "You want to create visual harmony in every room, and when you have too much stuff on display, it's crazy on the brain," McGurn says. So, rather than showing off all your keepsakes at once, put out only a few choice pieces at a time. Also, when you do put objects on display, including candlesticks, picture frames, even pillows, group them in odd numbers. "In pairs, you notice the difference," McGurn says. "Adding a third object creates a soothing compositional element."

6 Bring in nature

It's always nice to be reminded that there's a world outside our den, bath and kitchen. "Feeling disconnected from your natural environment causes anxiety," says McGurn, who recommends incorporating earth, wind, fire and water in every room. Hang window boxes outside, and display plants or fresh flowers inside to feel grounded. Open windows on opposite sides of the room to get fresh air moving in and dust moving out. Hang a picture of your favorite landscape on the wall. "Surrounding yourself with nature brings a sense of harmony," she says.

7 Engage all your senses

A room can look stunningly gorgeous, but if you're too scared to touch anything in it, the pretty factor is going to become old very quickly. A relaxing space appeals to senses other than sight.

Make every room a tactile experience by bringing in different textures. A soft chenille pillow will give you extra comfort. Lay lush wool rugs on hard floors, not only to pamper your feet but also to lessen sound vibrations. "Hard surfaces create echoes, which can be disorienting and stressful," McGurn says. Try varying rug textures from room to room, and use different scented candles to give each room a distinctive smell that corresponds to its mood.

8 Be open to change

Think about how revitalized you feel when you get a sexy new shade of lipstick for spring. Dress your home the way you dress yourself by making small changes to your space, using the seasons as your guide. Move one large piece of furniture (your couch or bed). If that's too much of a commitment, then swap out your bedspread, curtains or a rug to keep the room enlivened. "When you change your perspective, you notice different things in your house that you love. It rejuvenates your space, giving you a fresh viewpoint and engaging your mind and senses," McGurn says.

9 Choose colors that resonate

There is no right way to paint, McGurn says, but some colors can affect your mood. "Pastels offer a calming effect and are ideal for bedrooms," she says. In the spaces where you spend your morning, such as a bathroom or breakfast area, use a bright color, like yellow or green, to energize. Dining rooms tend to be more nurturing, enveloping and cozy, so try darker hues there. The bottom line: Choose colors that make sense to you. Ask yourself, How do I want to use this space? Then, What appeals to me?

10 Go with your gut

If something doesn't look or feel right, change it, period. You'll be living with it for a long time and you should never have to convince yourself you feel comfortable in your own home. You're the queen of your own castle. Rule on!

🕐 **GOT 10 MINUTES?**

Decipher your unique decorating style

Feathering your nest is easy when you have a sense of your interior design identity. Home decor magazines are filled with style-specific terms such as *21st century, retro* and *romantic*. Where do you fit in, and how can you use that knowledge to outfit your place? Find out below.

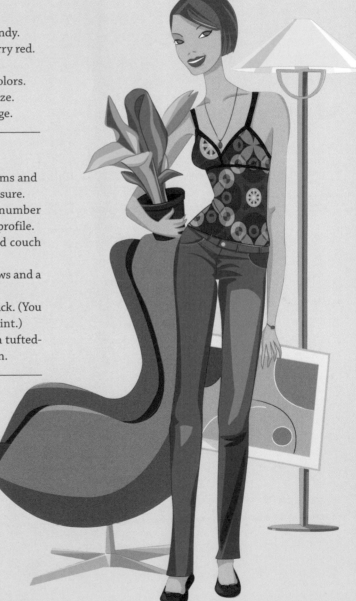

1 Your idea of a perfect color palette is...

A Cream accented by hunter green and burgundy.
B White with black and gray and a hint of cherry red.
C White punctuated by a fresh grass-green.
D Sunny yellow, with a touch of other floral colors.
E Rich taupe with hints of pale pink and bronze.
F Brilliant turquoise with chocolate and orange.

You chose _____

2 Your dream sofa is...

A A three-cushioned, skirted sofa with roll arms and a few matching throw pillows for good measure.
B A tight-backed, microsuede-upholstered number with squared-off arms and a sophisticated profile.
C A crisp, white, organic cotton–upholstered couch with a sturdy hardwood frame.
D A sink-right-in sofa with lots of throw pillows and a charming ticking-stripe slipcover.
E A plush fainting couch with a sexy, curved back. (You think it would look amazing in a leopard print.)
F A svelte sofa with gently sloped arms and a tufted-back upholstery in a mod geometric pattern.

You chose _____

3 You're hosting a dinner party but first you need to buy proper chairs. You head straight to...

A Your local department store, where you find a regal set of formal chairs with tie-on cushions.
B A cool boutique chain such as West Elm, where you choose a set of hip chairs.
C An online specialty retailer that sells chairs handcrafted from recycled wood.

D A mass retailer such as Pottery Barn for ladder-back chairs with a milk-paint finish and woven rush seats.

E An antique shop, where you rescue a handful of Victorian-style chairs with seats upholstered in silk.

F A vintage store that specializes in 1950s pine chairs. Their streamlined look feels *Jetsons,* yet comfy.

You chose _____

4 A picture is worth a thousand words. The one you decide to hang above your mantel says...

A You can't go wrong with a still-life painted in oil.

B Black-and-white silk-screen portraits are really in.

C You want to commune with nature by using a frameless mirror to reflect the landscape.

D You love folk art, especially farm scenes.

E A precious piece of vintage wallpaper in a gilded frame is every bit as interesting as a classic framed portrait.

F Long live Warhol! (Even a fake one will do.)

You chose _____

5 Your living room floor is too cold without a rug. It's time to shop, and you choose...

A An Oriental—eBay, here you come!

B A cut-pile rug with an eye-catching abstract pattern—or maybe just a solid.

C Something simple made of natural, woven sea grass or bamboo.

D A cozy, chenille braided rug.

E A simple Berber carpet.

F A funky flokati.

You chose _____

Score yourself and spot your style

MOSTLY As You're a traditionalist. You favor light-colored walls and darkly hued furniture.
Get the look instantly Paint trim and moldings in a color other than classic white to add a formal touch to your rooms. Shop for Chris Madden's furniture at JC Penney (JCPenney.com) or Restoration Hardware's own line (RestorationHardware.com).

MOSTLY Bs You're a modernist. You prefer sleek, sophisticated tables in glass, polished wood or medium-density fiberboard (known in the trade as MDF), as well as seating that's low in height and features clean, straight lines and exposed metal feet.
Get the look instantly Tidy up; mod rooms are neat. And add a hit of color in pale spaces as an accessory. Shop for Scandinavian 20th-century-inspired styles at Design Within Reach (DWR.com).

MOSTLY Cs You prefer the Zen vibe of organic minimalism that uses renewable materials such as bamboo, sea grass, recycled glass and salvaged wood.
Get the look instantly Lighten up rooms with grass rugs, organic cotton pillows and objects found in nature. Replace fiberglass with handmade furniture made of raw woods. Browse Thos. Moser Cabinetmakers (ThosMoser.com) or ABC Carpet & Home (ABCHome.com) to learn more.

MOSTLY Ds You're charmed by country-style decor.
Get the look instantly Swap in wicker chairs instead of armchairs, and hang a distressed vintage mirror or two. Be sure not to let the homespun vibe get too cutesy. Brainstorm ideas by looking at Rachel Ashwell Shabby Chic (ShabbyChic.com).

MOSTLY Es You're smitten with romantic interiors complete with overstuffed chairs and sofas and elegant, four-poster canopy beds.
Get the look instantly Upgrade your light fixtures. You can start small with bejeweled shades and shimmering crystal sconces, or you can go all out and hang an ornate chandelier. When shopping, get inspiration from Anthropologie (Anthropologie.com) and Barbara Barry (BarbaraBarry.com).

MOSTLY Fs Retro decor's mix of kitschy fabrics and funky furniture appeals to your playful side.
Get the look instantly Toss a few a geometric patterned pillows on your couch, or hang an iconic piece of art. Log on to Jonathan Adler (JonathanAdler.com) or Todd Oldham by La-Z-Boy (La-Z-Boy.com) for ideas.

🕐 GOT 15 MINUTES?

Simplify choosing a sofa Save time and stop stressing over one of the biggest furniture purchase you'll ever make with these straightforward shopping tricks.

Size up the situation

Before you buy a sofa, do one crucial thing, Alex Bates, senior vice president of product development for West Elm, advises: "Measure! Not only width, height and depth of the couch but all the entrances it will need to pass through to reach your room, as well as elevators and staircases and around banisters."

Envision your ideal arm

"The sofa arm is the main indicator of style," Bates says. A straight, rectangular-shaped Parson's arm is modern; a roll arm is traditional. Once you suss out the arm you like best, let that be your guide. You'll shave so much time off sofa shopping, you may even have the energy to move on to dining sets.

Kick back and relax

Because comfort is the most important thing when shopping for a couch, spend at least one minute sitting, slouching and lying down on your potential purchase. If you're a cuddler or a napper, remember: The lower the arm, the cozier curling up will be.

Scope out for screws

To get a quality sofa that will last, look for one with a solid hardwood frame joined with screws or dowels, not glue. "Tip it to see how it's made," Bates says. "Wiggle the arm. If it feels loose, move on. Floor models endure the same wear and tear you'll have at home."

🕐 GOT 10 MINUTES? Reclaim your Saturdays

Turn time-consuming weekend furniture hunts into daily 10-minute treats, minus the dust and cobwebs, by logging on to 1stDibs.com, where some of the country's best antique dealers post their hot finds.

⏱ GOT 8 MINUTES?
Zero in on your dream bed

Shopping for a bed frame doesn't have to be a nightmare. Prep with these time- and space-savers.

FIGHT SPRAWL Measure from the edges of your current bed to the nearest wall or piece of furniture. You need at least 3 feet to keep the space from feeling crowded. Now you know whether you should stick with your current size or choose a different one.

FIGURE OUT IF YOU NEED A LIFT When shopping, pause to lift the mattress; if the bed frame has slats or a platform, you can skip a box spring.

CONSIDER A BED THAT MULTITASKS If you're strapped for space, buy a bed with built-in drawers underneath for extra storage.

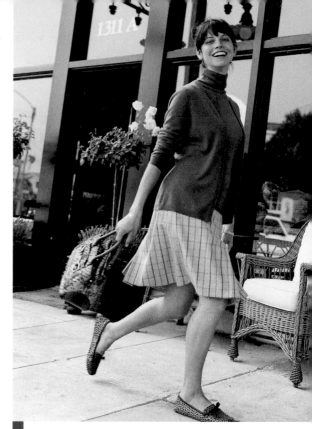

⏱ GOT 3 MINUTES?
Buy a mattress with confidence

Road test your future comfort zone with this superfast sleep-well check from Ira Fishman, vice president of merchandising for the northeast mattress chain Sleepy's: Lie down on the mattress. If you can stay in one position for three minutes, it's a keeper. If you need to adjust your position after 60 seconds, then it's not for you.

⏱ GOT 15 MINUTES?
Fix a mattress mistake

A mattress that's too soft can become instantly firmer if you slide a sheet of plywood underneath it. (Have it cut to size at your local lumberyard for a small fee.) A too-firm mattress, on the other hand, can be softened up with the help of a mattress topper made of memory foam or latex. For maximum benefits, try a 2-inch-thick topper (about $200).

⏱ GOT 15 MINUTES?
Think before you shop

Avoid buying things that don't fit into your decorating scheme by creating a design spec sheet. When you do, you'll stay on track rather than be swayed by a store's display. Here's how to do it:

1 Flip through magazines, and rip out images of rooms you like.

2 Lay them all on the floor, and quickly scan the pages for similarities. They could be the wall color, accessories, a light source or the shape of the furniture.

3 Find what you love the most on each page, and cut it out as best you can.

4 On a blank piece of paper, tape or glue favorite items to create a rudimentary collage of your dream room.

5 Bring it with you when you're shopping for rugs, furniture, paint and more, and refer to it when making choices. Can you picture the item you're debating buying in this setting? If not, pass it by.

🕐 GOT 15 MINUTES?

Devise a color scheme

Design a perfect palette without worry with these easy-to-follow, decorator-approved guidelines.

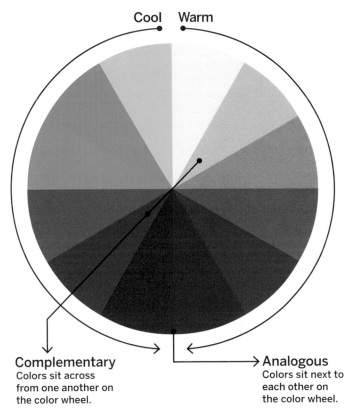

Cool   Warm

Complementary
Colors sit across from one another on the color wheel.

Analogous
Colors sit next to each other on the color wheel.

1 Go monochromatic. Stick with your favorite hue—let's say it's blue—and use a range of different shades within the blue family to keep things interesting. Robin's egg blue, turquoise and cobalt are all related, and together they make for a nicely layered palette.

2 Consider complementary colors such as blue and orange or purple and green. Choose one shade to dominate, and make the other the accent. When two complementary colors are used equally, it's overpowering and best saved for sports teams.

3 Follow the analogous color rule: Colors that adjoin each other along the wheel are easy to blend and almost always result in a harmonious overall look. Let yourself have fun. Pick two to four of these colors, then apply them liberally to create a scheme.

🕐 GOT 15 MINUTES?

Learn how to pick and pair any pattern

Mix and match patterns using these reliable rules.

Keep colors in the same family. A good rule of thumb is to make sure the patterns share at least two colors in common; three is ideal. But the shades don't have to be an identical match.

Pay attention to scale. Opt for different patterns that are of similar scale, such as small- and medium-sized prints or large and extra large ones. Doing this leaves a multiple-pattern scheme looking pulled together, not random.

Do a background check. If you want to play it safe, place patterns against a solid white background and let them take center stage. For a more dramatic effect, isolate colors within your patterns and use them on your walls.

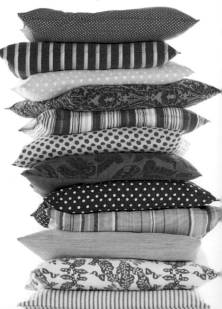

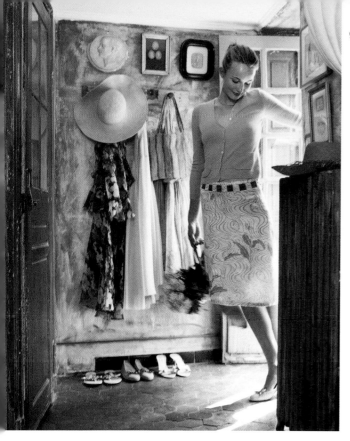

⏱ GOT 15 MINUTES?
Decorate with bold color fearlessly

Banish what-if-I-hate-it worries with this no-fail tip from Julia M. Williams of Julia Williams Interiors in West Linn, Oregon. Take 15 minutes to paint patches of different colors in several places around a room or on foam core boards, which you can throw away when you're done. Live with the shade for at least a full 24 hours before you make your decision. Notice how the colors behave throughout the day as the natural light changes. Afterward, you'll feel more confident about your choice.

⏱ GOT 15 MINUTES? Try accent colors

You can spice up your pad with minimal effort by painting strategically chosen accents in different rooms. Follow this cheat sheet:

IN THE KITCHEN
- Paint the inside of your cabinet doors.
- Switch boring cabinet hardware for painted knobs.
- Stock up on colorful dinner and flatware, and use it everyday.

IN THE LIVING ROOM
- Treat a ceiling or floor as a fifth wall by painting it.
- Glue a bright fabric inside a sheer lamp shade. The color will show through when the light is on.

IN THE BEDROOM
- Hang a vibrant set of sheer curtains to create a refreshing wash of color through a room.
- Add a splashy dust ruffle for a surprise ending.

⏱ GOT 1 MINUTE?
Discover the safest pattern

So you want something interesting in your room, but you shy away from using a big, bold pattern? Never fear. Choose a fabric with a pronounced texture. For instance, corduroy ribs look like stripes and behave that way when they cover throw pillows, even if the fabric is a solid color.

⏱ GOT 1 MINUTE?
Use color to define size

Bedrooms and dining rooms benefit from an element of intimacy, but this mood can be hard to achieve in a space that's too wide open, such as a loft, for instance. Remedy the problem by picking a warm color for the walls—reds, oranges and yellows—which will make them appear to come forward, so the space seems more enclosed. The opposite works for small spaces, too. The eye perceives cool, pale shades as receding, so tiny spaces seem airy.

⊕ GOT 15 MINUTES?

Rearrange your living room in a flash

Inject instant ambience with this floor plan, which is so versatile it works for almost every living room. It's courtesy of interior designer Maxwell Gillingham-Ryan.

Designate a home for your TV

Place the TV and media stand along the wall facing the couch for easy viewing, but make sure it doesn't dominate the room.

Master your mantel

Arrange decorative items such as vases or candlesticks off-center and to the left on a mantel or table. The asymmetry is less predictable and more pleasing to the eye.

Hang petite pictures on stairs

The secret is to arrange the pictures in relationship to each other, not in relationship to each individual step.

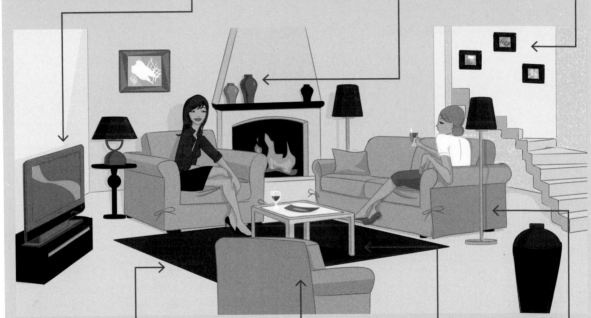

Frame the room

Rugs define a room. If you have a light floor, use a dark rug to define the social space. If you have a dark floor, pick a light rug to make the area seem more expansive.

Set the scene

You should have at least three points of seating—for example, a circle composed of one sofa and two chairs facing it. You're creating a social setting, so people come right in and start talking.

Create focus with a coffee table

"People leave the center open because they think it makes the room look larger," Gillingham-Ryan explains, "but it leaves it seeming uncentered."

Let there be light

Follow the three-points-of-light rule to create warmth all over: Put a lamp on either side of the sofa and one by a chair. Or two by chairs and one by the sofa.

⏱ GOT 15 MINUTES?
Create the perfect composition

Grouping artwork and photos is easy if you treat the cluster as one big piece of art. Lay everything on the floor, and experiment with various arrangements. When you hit on a composition that works for you, identify the centerpiece. Hang it first, then adjust the other items around it following your desired format.

⏱ GOT 5 MINUTES?
Fake an extra window

There's a reason homes with southern exposure are priced at a premium: Natural light makes your place seem bigger. It's also mood lifting, so try this get-happy trick: Find your brightest window and hang a mirror on a wall perpendicular to it (not opposite it). "It will bounce the sun's rays into every part of the room," multiplying the light, McGurn says. Now that's something to smile about.

⏱ GOT 10 MINUTES?
Hang any picture at the ideal height

Save time putting up pictures by following what Gillingham-Ryan calls the 57-inches-on-center rule. "This is gallery height," he explains. "It seems low, but it's actually natural eye level." The process is easy: Simply measure 57 inches from the floor and place the center of your picture over that point. This technique ensures that your pictures, whatever their size, will have midpoints in sync throughout the room.

⏱ GOT 10 MINUTES?
Style smarter bookshelves

Think of your bookshelf as a pyramid of your intellect. Place heavy tomes, oversize photo albums and storage boxes on the bottom. The books you reach for often should live in the middle, around eye level. It's fine to mix and match hardcover and softcover if you organize by author, though organizing by color looks better. Lastly, place a delicate objet d'art on top. It will be safely out of reach and will draw the eye upward, making the room seem more expansive.

⏱ GOT 6 MINUTES?
View your passions in a new way

DISPLAYING A COLLECTION is a great way to surround yourself with the things you love. Here are two no-fail tips for pulling it off with ease.

FIND THE COMMONALITY "The fun of collections is showing off their subtle similarities and their differences," Gillingham-Ryan says. If the objects have different heights, different textures and different shapes, then they should all be the same color or at least in the same color family. If they're different colors and textures, then they should be the same shape.

KEEP IT TOGETHER Always group a collection together. If you display yours in shadow boxes, it can even double as art. The worst way to display a collection is to spread it throughout a house. Seeing the same thing over and over can get relentless and looks campy, not sophisticated.

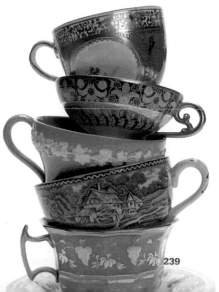

239

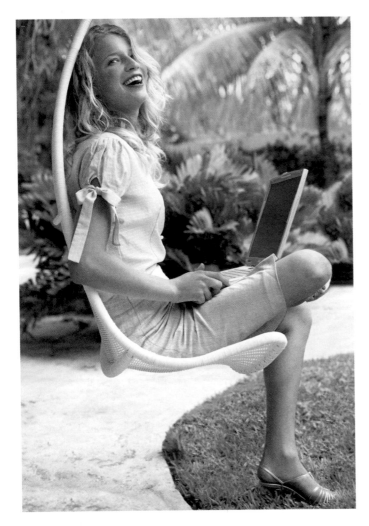

⏱ GOT 10 MINUTES?
Prep to interview a potential decorator

To ensure your first home-decor choice, the decorator, is the right one, screen him before you commit to hiring him. Use this list of suggested questions from decorators Laura Smolen of SR Hughes in Tulsa, Oklahoma, and Brooke Gomez of Gomez Associates in New York City.

- How long have you been in the business?
- Where did you study design, and what degrees do you have?
- What types of houses or apartments have you designed, and where are they located?
- What's your schedule like? What amount of your time will you be able to devote to my project, and for how long?
- How are you paid? (Most designers charge a retainer, an hourly fee and a markup of 30 to 35 percent on furniture and accessories. But designers purchase your pieces wholesale—typically 33⅓ percent less than consumers pay—so the difference usually evens out in the end.)
- What would you estimate this project is going to cost me?
- How do you see the furniture I already own fitting into the new design scheme?
- Could I see a sample contract?

⏱ GOT 1 MINUTE?
Rely on word of mouth

When it comes to finding an interior designer, drop in on your favorite home decor stores and ask for recommendations. Using a local decorator is convenient, and you can meet easily and visit the homes she's done in your town.

⏱ GOT 2 MINUTES?
Rein in the spending spree

IF YOU'RE ON a budget (aren't we all?), remember these two easy ways to keep your decorator on track when it comes to expenses. **ASK HER TO DO THE PROCESS IN STAGES** Many professionals will go room by room, pausing to let your cash reserves build. **FIND A MORE EXERIENCED DESIGNER** An interior decorator who has had more than 10 years in the business can tell you authoritatively when to scrimp and where to invest; she'll also have a Rolodex full of contractors, as well as perspective on brands and knowledge of which last and which don't.

⏱ GOT 10 MINUTES? Learn decorating lingo

When a decorator opens her mouth or you visit a home store, does it sound as if you're hearing a foreign language? Are you baffled by the terms thrown around, like *baffle* (the shapes on down comforters preventing the filling from bunching)? Add the following design terms to your lexicon and start talking the talk.

Baluster A column that supports a stair handrail

Bolster A cylindrical pillow most often flanking an armless sofa or used as part of a bedding ensemble, either decoratively or to prop up the neck

Cabriole leg An S-shaped furniture leg that mimics the shape of an animal's hind leg, a staple of Queen Anne–style furniture

Chaise lounge From the French for "long chair," an upholstered piece of seating meant for reclining

Chinoiserie A Western interpretation of Chinese decoration, it usually takes the form of hand-painted pagodas or landscapes painted on furniture.

Cornice A decorative, horizontal molding located at the top of the wall and often used to conceal window treatment fixtures

Credenza Also called a sideboard or buffet, a wooden storage chest found in dining rooms

Damask A fabric with a tone-on-tone quality usually featuring figured stripes or jacquard, an ornate pattern weave

Design library A list of all the types of resources interior designers have that are available only to the trade

Étagère A freestanding unit with open shelving used to display or to store objects

Gooseneck spout A type of faucet popular in kitchens, it has a curved U-shape and a high arc.

Matelasse From the French for cushioned, this fabric is quilted and double-woven with a raised surface often used on bedspreads, throws and slipcovers.

Parquet Geometrically patterned wood inlays used primarily in flooring

Puddle A style of hanging drapes with an extra 6 to 8 inches of fabric to pool on the floor

Physical vapor deposition (PVD) The process by which a colored finish is bonded onto the metal of a plumbing fixture. Once bonded, the color is scratch- and tarnish-resistant.

Settee A wide armchair; it is generally upholstered but has no loose cushions and seats two.

Subway tile This ceramic tile gets its name from its resemblance to tiles used on the walls of subway stations; it's often used in bathrooms.

Swag A window treatment consisting of loose material draped over a curtain rod

Thread count The number of horizontal and vertical threads per square inch; generally, the higher the thread count, the softer the fabric.

Vessel sink A bowl-shaped sink that appears to be sitting atop a counter but is actually plumbed in; it's used mostly in the bathroom.

Vitreous china Ceramic that's fired at a very high temperature and glazed, making it virtually impervious to stains. Brands such as Kohler and American Standard often use this material for kitchens and baths. It is also called porcelain enamel.

Wainscoting Wood paneling that's applied to the lower half of a wall and finished with a piece of horizontal molding known as a chair rail—so called because it's typically level with the top of a chair and prevents the chair from scuffing the wall.

Widespread lavatory faucet A faucet whose hot- and cold-water handles are unattached to its spout, unlike a centerset faucet, whose handles and spout are connected to a central base.

⏱ GOT 15 MINUTES (OR LESS)?

Clean and declutter
Sure, you'd love to carve out a day for a deep-down scrub, but who has the time? Tackle your domestic trouble spots bit by bit with this tip sheet.

(15 MIN) Dust delicate items
When dusting valuables, you want something light like a feather duster; but the sad truth is feather dusters don't eliminate dust; they brush it from one surface to another. A better bet is a Swiffer duster. Dust clings to its fibers because the cloth is electrostatically treated, says Barbara Roche Fierman, owner of New York's Little Elves, a cleaning service in New York City. Use a Swiffer with an extendable handle to clean paintings, chandeliers (be sure the chandelier has been turned off and is cool) and any hard-to-reach item.

(1 MIN) Sniffleproof your pillow
Pillows may contain up to 16 species of allergy-triggering fungi, so run your synthetic one through the washing machine (hot-water cycle) and dryer every three months. Once it's dry, encase it in an allergy-proof cover (available at bedding stores). It blocks particles like dirt, sweat and skin, which dust mites thrive on. (Cover down pillows as well.) And the next time you make the bed, open your windows first. According to the journal *Environmental Science & Technology,* making the bed stirs up dust that can cause an allergy attack.

(8 MIN) Degunk your coffeemaker
Once a month, pour a cup of undiluted white vinegar into the water reservoir and turn on the pot. When it completes its cycle, discard the vinegar and run a cup of water through the reservoir. Rinse the pot thoroughly afterward to eliminate any residual aftertaste. Your morning brew will taste better.

(15 MIN) Remove mildew from tile
Keep air flowing from a fan or open window and you'll reduce the likelihood of mold recurring in the bathroom. If it's already there, use any kind of bathroom detergent and a nylon bristle brush. Brushes that use natural hair aren't as durable, and you have to replace them more often. Choose a brush with stiff nylon bristles around the periphery and soft ones in the middle. The hard bristles loosen mold in tough-to-reach nooks; the softer ones massage the gunk out of hard surfaces.

(15 MIN) Freshen your fridge
Move over, baking soda. If you want your refrigerator to smell refreshingly clean, try this quirky trick from Fierman: Leave a container of used coffee grinds in the back of your fridge. The grinds absorb icky odors without giving your fridge the aroma of your local coffeehouse.

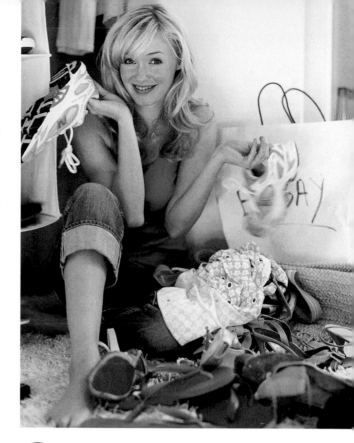

2 MIN Make a nice entrance

One reason we sigh over the rooms in decorating magazines is that they never contain the piles of stuff that haunt us in real life. To achieve that spare look, use this tip from Elaine Griffin, an interior designer in New York City: Put one good-looking bin and a desktop tray by the front door for mail and keys. Use another near a staircase to collect items destined for other floors. Both items will help you master the paradox of keeping things hidden and accessible.

5 MIN Purge painlessly

Jen M. R. Doman, owner of Get It Together!, an organizing service in Brooklyn, New York, offers four simple questions that will help you know what to keep and what to finally bid adieu to.

- When you look at the item, does it bring up unpleasant memories of a tough time? Sentimental keepsakes should promote feelings of happiness, not regret.
- Do you have a home for it? If you don't immediately envision the spot where you think it belongs, it's a clue that you may no longer need it.
- Is there someone else (a friend or family member, even a charity) who would enjoy the item more than you do? If so, put it on your giveaway pile.
- When did you last use it? If it has been more than three months and it is not a seasonal item (such as your Christmas tree stand), chances are, you can do without it and not even notice.

15 MIN Straighten up for surprise guests

Drop-in guests are always fun; what isn't is worrying about the state of your house in the 15 minutes you have before they arrive. Try this speedy clean-up tip the next time a friend calls to ask if she can stop by. First, attack the areas she'll see as soon as she walks in so the house gives the impression of cleanliness. If you have time, vacuum up any unsightly dust bunnies. Clear counters of clutter by simply putting whatever was on top in a cabinet underneath and placing dishes in the sink. Throw whatever else is lying around into a tote bag in a closet devoted expressly to clutter—not the coat closet, which guests are bound to see if they hang up their coats. Light a scented candle in the foyer for ambience, and say phew!

1 MIN Make goody bags

Purging can be a good reason for a party. Gather unwanted items into gift bags and invite pals over for a giveaway brunch, suggests Judi Culbertson, a professional organizer in New York City. After mimosas, they take their pick and lighten your load.

1 MIN Establish a giveaway table

SELF staffers are inundated with props from shoots, so we have giveaway tables on which we place unwanted items for other coworkers to take. Why not do the same at home? Designate a space for stuff you don't want so friends can pick up freebies. (The only downside is you may have more surprise guests!)

1 MIN Smell organized

When you don't have time to actually tidy up, a clean-scented candle can work wonders in making your space feel pulled together. After cooking, light food-scented candles—lemon, lime or pomegranate in the kitchen. Try green tea or jasmine in the living room or a spalike scent—eucalyptus or sage —in the bathroom. You'll feel Zen with the flick of a match.

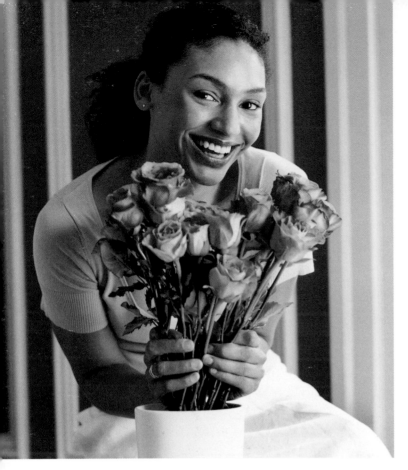

GOT 15 MINUTES?
Make a more fetching centerpiece

Two winning ways to create stunning arrangements:

1 CLUSTER YOUR CONTAINERS Put a single blossom into several glass bottles, slender drinking glasses or bud vases of different heights. Be sure to vary the height of the flowers—have some fall right at the lip; stand others taller and add a leaf here and there. Arrange them together on a tray, or run them along the center of a table with votive candles.

2 MASS ONE TYPE OF BLOOM Buy a large quantity of a single flower, cut the stems to varying lengths (aim to make the tallest flowers one third higher than the height of the vase) and place them in a classic trumpet vase. Start around the outside lip of the container and work your way in. The stems will interlock and stay securely in place.

GOT 5 MINUTES?
Add fragrance with flowers

Whether you're choosing flowers for indoors or for your garden, let blooms lead you by the nose. From Mary Cashman, senior horticulturist for White Flower Farm in Litchfield, Connecticut:

STRONG SCENT
You smell these from a distance:
- Lavender, in full sun, can be quite fragrant; on a cloudy day, the scent isn't as strong.
- Gardenia
- Jasmine
- Lilac
- Narcissus
- Oriental lily and trumpet lily
- Peony

MEDIUM SCENT
You smell these standing close by:
- Roses—old varieties and David Austin hybrids are generally the most fragrant
- Cherry branches
- Dianthus
- Heliotrope
- Lily of the valley
- Phlox
- Sweet pea
- Sweet violet

LIGHT SCENT
You smell these only next to your nose:
- Echinacea smell strongest in morning and evening.
- Chrysanthemum
- Geranium
- Iris
- Monarda
- Poppies
- Snapdragon
- Sweet alyssum
- Tulip

GOT 4 MINUTES?
Try a new vase

Don't limit yourself to the same old containers. A few to try instead:
- Old silver trophies
- Pitchers, creamers, teapots
- Milk bottles or mason jars
- Watering cans or old sap buckets
- Silver mint julep cups
- Bowls (a flower frog holds stems)

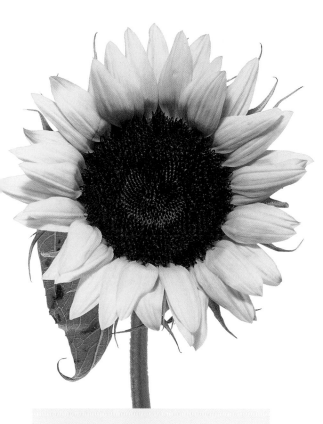

⏱ GOT 9 MINUTES?
Help fresh flowers last longer

Follow these rules so your bouquets kabloom before they go kaput.

● Get flowers from a reliable source. Grocery stores, while convenient, often do not have the freshest flowers.

● Strip away any leaves that will be below the water line in the vase—they produce bacteria that kills buds faster.

● For woody branches, make three cuts vertically about an inch up the stems to help them drink. Contrary to popular belief, you shouldn't smash woody stems; it hurts their molecular structure.

● Put a floral food such as Floralife or Chrysal into the water.

● Keep flowers in as cool a spot as possible but avoid placing them next to air conditioners or anywhere with extreme temperature fluctuations.

● Change the water daily or every other day. Put an intricate arrangement under the tap and add fresh water until you've flushed out all the old water. Recut or pluck out any wilting blossoms. When flowers start to fade, cut down the stems and transfer the flowers to a shorter vase; doing this can revive them.

⏱ GOT 5 MINUTES?
Send a perennial favorite

Instead of giving someone cut flowers, consider choosing a flowering plant like an azalea, which can be planted in the spring and enjoyed for years to come.

⏱ GOT 5 MINUTES?
Buy naturally long-lasting cut flowers

Look beyond the obvious carnations and mums to these petals that keep on giving.

Allium	Lilies
Alstroemeria	Lisianthus
Baby's breath	Orchids
Birds-of-paradise	Star-of-Bethlehem
Ginger	(including
Gladiolus	*Ornithogalum*
Godetia	*arabicum*)
Heliconia	Sunflowers

⏲ GOT 15 MINUTES?
Plan a stress-free party

Lauren Purcell, SELF deputy editor and cofounder of PurcellSisters.com, a party planning site, explains how to prep in a few minutes a day.

SEVEN DAYS BEFORE Make a list of what you need to buy.

SIX DAYS BEFORE Buy hors d'oeuvres and freeze them.

FIVE DAYS BEFORE Drop in on your local party store to stock up on supplies—napkins, cups, decorations, candles.

FOUR DAYS BEFORE Tidy up your home; stash extra toilet paper in the bathroom. Give your medicine cabinet and vanity a once-over and make them look neat.

THREE DAYS BEFORE Wipe down all serving trays and bowls. Make a list of anything you still need to get.

TWO DAYS BEFORE Set up a buffet table.

ONE DAY BEFORE Buy mixers, lemons and limes. Call a liquor store and arrange to have beverages delivered.

DAY OF PARTY Place candles around the room. Open and reclose tonic and soda to prevent carbonation explosions. Get a pedicure. While there make your to do list, and remember, if your feet are happy, everything else will be, too.

⏲ GOT 3 MINUTES?
Appoint a 6:30 friend

Regardless of how well prepared you are, time flies when you're party prepping. Ask a friend to come at 6:30 to do all those small but important things you thought you'd have time to do but don't. Avoid asking cohosts or boyfriends. They'll have already been doing their fair share and will need to get ready as well.

⏲ GOT 1 MINUTE?
Determine how much ice you need

Purcell likes to say, "Ice is to parties as gas is to cars." You just can't run one without it. And when you use it all up, everything grinds to a halt. For a party at which you will serve the drinks on the rocks, calculate a pound of ice per guest. If ice counts as an ingredient, as in a mojito, calculate 2 pounds per person. Given those quantities, go out and buy it. Look for ice with the International Packaged Ice Association seal; it's the most pure.

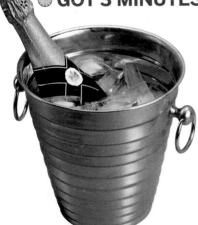

⏲ GOT 3 MINUTES? Pop open bubbly

Open Champagne fearlessly.
● Make sure the bottle is chilled.
● Open the foil capsule; unwind the wire hood, but leave it on to make the cork easier to hold.
● Wrap a towel around the bottle neck to improve grip.
● With your right hand, hold the cork in place. Turn the bottle with your left hand.
● After two full turns of the bottle you should hear a pop. Voilà! Champagne, anyone?

GOT 15 MINUTES?
Cut down on your kitchen time or avoid it completely

IF YOU HAVE more money than time, dial in hors d'oeuvres with these quick and easy picks:

JAPANESE Sushi rolls are a favorite. Also try edamame, which can be served in bowls, yakitori (grilled chicken skewers) and shrimp shumai, which you can easily pick up with a toothpick.

CHINESE Serve spring rolls (but not egg rolls, which are difficult to cut into individual pieces) as well as shrimp toasts.

MEXICAN You can never go wrong with chips, spicy salsa and fresh guacamole. You can also try quesadillas; ask for them whole, then cut them into bite-size wedges at home. Another tip: Look over the menu to find tiny versions of hearty favorites—for instance, empanadas are also served as an appetizer, called empanaditas.

GREEK Start with stuffed grape leaves and spana-kopita (phyllo triangles filled with spinach and feta cheese). Then get an assortment of dips, and be sure to ask for lots of extra pita.

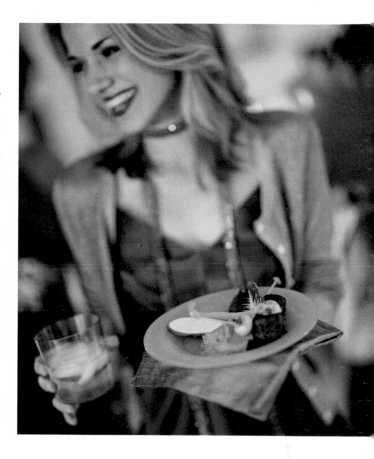

GOT 15 MINUTES?
Mingle gracefully

The trick to making clever conversation while multitasking as hostess is to arm yourself with a tray of hors d'oeuvres, says Purcell, who is the coauthor of *Cocktail Parties, Straight Up!* (Wiley). She who holds the tray must keep moving. As you navigate the room, you get to give each guest a dollop of personal attention and offer her food. People will seek you and your tray, which allows conversational groups to shift. It also offers you an excellent opportunity to make introductions. Friends feel taken care of, and you feel as if you're connecting with the party rather than being stuck in the kitchen. Spot a shy partygoer? Hand the tray to her, and let her mix with guests.

GOT 3 MINUTES?
Don't be surprised by your guests' behavior

PREPARE FOR THE inevitable by anticipating what always happens at every party.

Guests will congregate in the kitchen. It's a magnet because it feels comfortable and casual. Let them camp out by serving them the crudités, or give yourself space by sending them out with hors d'oeuvres to feed the party.

Someone will spill or break something. Keep wipes on hand and your DustBuster charged, and remind the spiller or breaker that it's not a party until you hear a crash.

Friends will look in your medicine cabinet. Hide the hemorrhoid cream.

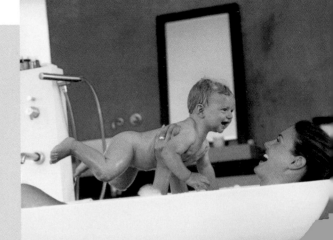

🕐 GOT 5 MINUTES?

Learn how to make each room green

Check out this list of home appliances you use every day that you could easily upgrade to eco-friendly status. In general, an Energy Star appliance may cost more initially. But if you do decide to buy one, it should pay for itself in five years or less, and it will continue to save you money each passing year.

THE KITCHEN

● **Refrigerator** Upgrading a fridge bought in 1990 would save enough power to light your home for up to four months. When choosing your fridge, remember that ones with freezers on top use up to 15 percent less energy than the side-by-side kind.

● **Dishwasher** When shopping, look for a dishwasher with an air-dry cycle; it dries dishes with a fan rather than a heating coil, thereby using less power.

THE BATHROOM

The Environmental Protection Agency introduced a WaterSense label in the fall of 2006 to educate consumers about water conservation and water-efficient products for indoor and outdoor use. Look for it on toilets, faucets, showerheads and landscape-irrigation systems.

● **Toilet** Toilets installed before 1992 use 3.5 to 7 gallons of water per flush. New high-efficiency toilets use less than 1.3 gallons per flush and save you $90 a year.

● **Showerhead** A low-flow showerhead feels exactly like a regular showerhead, uses less energy to heat water and can save you up to $50 a year.

THE LAUNDRY ROOM

● **Washing machine** If your washer was bought before 1994, you may want to upgrade. Today's efficient washers use only 18 to 25 gallons of water per load compared with 40 gallons in a standard model. Plus, most Energy Star units now squeeze more water from clothes in the spin cycle. The shorter drying time that results saves energy and is gentler on your clothes.

● **Dryers** Surprisingly, dryers old and new use the same amount of energy, and there are no Energy Star–labeled dryers. You can still conserve, however, by purchasing a unit with a moisture sensor that detects when clothes are dry and shuts off automatically. Or better yet, dry your delicates and casual clothes on a rack indoors or on a line outside.

THE BASEMENT

● **Water heater** Be sure your water heater has an insulating jacket to bring down costs. When the time comes to replace it, choose one that has a higher energy factor rating.

THROUGHOUT YOUR HOME

● **Air-conditioning** You should replace a room air conditioner that's more than 10 years old; newer models can save up to 50 percent more energy and nearly $20 a year. Choose the unit with the highest energy efficiency ratio available. Energy Star requirements range from 9.4 to 10.8, depending on the size of the unit, but some units can have an EER as high as 12. If your central air-conditioning system is older than 10 years, replacing it will save you 20 percent in costs. Energy efficient systems have a seasonal energy efficiency ratio (SEER) rating that starts at 13, with the highest going up to 19, so select the one that comes closest to that number.